THE NEW RULES OF LIFTING

THE NEW RULES OF LIFTING

Six Basic Moves for Maximum Muscle

Lou Schuler and
Alwyn Cosgrove

AVERY
A MEMBER OF PENGUIN GROUP (USA) INC.
NEW YORK

Published by the Penguin Group

Penguin Group (USA) Inc., 375 Hudson Street, New York, New York 10014, USA ·
Penguin Group (Canada), 90 Eglinton Avenue East, Suite 700, Toronto, Ontario M4P 2Y3, Canada (a division of
Pearson Canada Inc.) · Penguin Books Ltd, 80 Strand, London WC2R 0RL, England · Penguin Ireland,
25 St Stephen's Green, Dublin 2, Ireland (a division of Penguin Books Ltd) · Penguin Group (Australia), 250
Camberwell Road, Camberwell, Victoria 3124, Australia (a division of Pearson Australia Group Pty Ltd) · Penguin
Books India Pvt Ltd, 11 Community Centre, Panchsheel Park, New Delhi–110 017, India · Penguin Group (NZ),
67 Apollo Drive, Rosedale, North Shore 0632, New Zealand (a division of Pearson New Zealand Ltd) · Penguin
Books (South Africa) (Pty) Ltd, 24 Sturdee Avenue, Rosebank, Johannesburg 2196, South Africa

Penguin Books Ltd, Registered Offices:
80 Strand, London WC2R 0RL, England

First trade paperback edition 2009
Copyright © 2006 by Lou Schuler and Alwyn Cosgrove

Most Avery books are available at special quantity discounts for bulk purchase for sales promotions, premiums,
fund-raising, and educational needs. Special books or book excerpts also can be created to fit specific needs.
For details, write Penguin Group (USA) Inc. Special Markets, 375 Hudson Street, New York, NY 10014.

The Library of Congress has catalogued the hardcover as follows:

Schuler, Lou.
The new rules of lifting: six basic moves for maximum muscle / Lou Schuler and Alwyn Cosgrove.
p.   cm.
Includes bibliographical references and index.
ISBN 1-58333-238-3
1. Weight lifting.   2. Bodybuilding.   3. Muscle strength.   I. Cosgrove, Alwyn.   II. Title.
GV546.3.S37   2005   2005053015
613.7'13—dc22

ISBN 978-1-58333-338-9 (paperback edition)

Printed in the United States of America
7   9   10   8   6

BOOK DESIGN BY TANYA MAIBORODA

Acknowledgments

I COULD NEVER OFFER enough thanks to the many strength coaches, trainers, re-searchers, and all-around gurus who taught me everything I know about exercise (and helped me unlearn what I thought I knew). At the top of the list is Alwyn Cos-grove, who has more creative and counterintuitive training ideas than anyone I've ever met. I also have to single out Mike Mejia, my coauthor and colleague for many years, who introduced me to Alwyn; and Stuart McGill, Ph.D., whose studies, lec-tures, and books (including *Ultimate Back Fitness and Performance*) inform almost every chapter of *The New Rules of Lifting*.

Someday I'll build a shrine to my agent, David Black, and to my editor, Megan Newman, a fellow lifter who was the first to see the potential in this project and worked so hard to make it happen. Thanks also to Rebecca Behan at Avery, Mark Cohen and Mike Caruso at *Men's Journal*, Adam Campbell, John Williams, Jeremy Katz, Mitch Mandel, Susan Eugster, and Matt Neumaier.

My wife, Kimberly Heinrichs, had to repeat the phrase, "Be quiet—Dad's work-ing!" more than any human should have to utter any four-word sequence. If not for her, this book would be scheduled for release sometime in 2010.

Last, I want to thank my older brother, G.O., who first got me hooked on lifting. He taught me that muscles are cool, and that hard work is life's great equalizer. I still think muscles are cool and, although it took me a while, I eventually came around to the idea that good, hard, honest work beats the hell out of the alternatives. A life without excuses is truly the good life.

L.S.

THANK YOU TO MY COACH, Derek Campbell—still, in my opinion, the greatest coach the world has ever seen—for being my mentor, my coach, and my friend. To all the athletes and clients who have trusted me with their bodies, thank you for believing in me. To my friends, colleagues, and teammates over the years, thank you for pushing me to new levels. Thanks to Lou Schuler, who first recognized my ideas on training and let me share them with the world via *Men's Health* magazine. To the team at Results Fitness, thank you for allowing me to test my theories on you. Thanks to my dad, who taught me that you can do whatever you set your mind to. Thank you to Rachel—my wife, my life partner, and my soul mate—for believing in me more than anyone else.

And thank you to my mum, who never got the chance to see the lessons she instilled in me take root and bear fruit. This book is for you.

A.C.

Contents

Introduction: The Truth of the Matter

LET ME TELL YOU about something I invented. I call it "weight lifting." Maybe you've heard it called "strength training," or "resistance training," or even "bodybuilding." But when I made it up in my basement, I called it weight lifting.

Are your B.S. detectors buzzing? Good. If they aren't, put in fresh batteries and read that paragraph again.

I want you to read everything in this book with at least a little skepticism. That may seem like a strange thing to ask of someone who's just paid real money for my book. But it's important, for two reasons:

1. If you read with the idea that maybe I'm not being completely truthful, you'll read more carefully, and that's exactly what I want.
2. Once you've read this with something less than fawning admiration of every sentence my fingers type, you'll be able to read future articles and books with the same raised eyebrow. (Although you'll have to buy my next book, *The Drooping-Face Cure*, to get my exclusive eyebrow-raising exercises.)

And then my work will be finished, and I can spend some time with my kids before they grow their own B.S. detectors and turn them on me at the dinner table.

SO . . . WHAT'S ACTUALLY IN THE BOOK?

If you've followed my career, you know I've written a bunch of books on exercise and diet. If you haven't followed my career . . . well, I've written a bunch of books on exercise and diet. (Thanks for letting me clear that up.) Starting with *The Testosterone Advantage Plan* and continuing with *The* Men's Health *Home Workout Bible* and *The Book of Muscle,* I've had two goals: Show guys how to build muscle and lose fat safely and effectively, and find new ways to make it more fun and interesting.

The book I haven't written—the book that I don't think anyone has written—is the one that takes everything we know about building a stronger, leaner, more muscular, more powerful, and longer-lasting body . . . and boils it down to its simplest, easiest-to-remember, and easiest-to-apply elements.

To accomplish that, Alwyn and I had to strip away everything about strength training that's useless, redundant, and even dangerous. As you read *New Rules,* you'll be surprised at how much of that stuff is out there. We'll show you, for example, a back-strengthening machine that actually causes spinal injuries. We'll explain why some accepted wisdom in the iron culture is false ("slow lifts are safe, fast lifts are dangerous"—we beat the snot out of that one) and why most of what people do in gyms fails to get them to their goals.

I think that what Alwyn and I present here is a new paradigm in exercise. Or, more accurately, the revival of an old paradigm. We want you to think of weight lifting in terms of how it changes your body's abilities, as opposed to how it changes your body's appearance. Trust me, *form will follow function.* Coordinated, useful muscles will still turn heads at the beach. But they'll also help you live longer and better.

Look at it this way: When my coauthors and I published *Testosterone Advantage,* many readers had no idea that low-fat diets were a bad idea for the guy who wants a leaner, more muscular physique. We showed the benefits of healthy fats—and of increased protein intake and controlled carbohydrate consumption. Since then, the nutrition universe has tilted 90 degrees, and the junk-food industry now touts its "low-carb" choices, whereas just a few years ago "low fat" was the most important selling point. (Junk food is still junk food, whether it's low fat or low carb, but that's a chapter for a different book.)

We also advocated strength training as the ideal fitness tool, whether you're trying to bulk up, slim down, or just look better at the same size. That, too, was surprising to many readers, who'd been told for years that if they wanted to lose weight, they had to lace up those running shoes. (To their credit, everyone was clear about the need to lift weights to *gain* muscular weight.)

Now, I think, it's time to redefine weight lifting itself. It's time to take out the exercises—most of them, actually—that do nothing to improve your ability to move better. It's time to add in the exercises that give you the most benefit in the least time.

Here's how I'll lay it out:

Part 1 of *New Rules* looks at strength training as *a series of elemental movements, with real-life applications.* Then I'll show how those movements become muscle-building exercises that, once mastered, become parts of routines that will evolve and adapt to your changing interests and abilities.

Part 2 shows you how training programs are constructed, and explains the other elements that go into a solid workout program. We'll show you how to warm up before lifting, how to increase or maintain your flexibility, and how to incorporate sports or endurance-building exercise.

Part 3 shows you the exercises derived from the six basic movement patterns—squat, deadlift, lunge, push, pull, twist.

Part 4 is the nitty-gritty—the programs created by Alwyn. These workouts are modular, meaning that you can mix or match them for different goals—bigger muscles, fat loss, improved strength, or a bit of each. (I know it sounds like we've just complicated things, but trust us: The modular system is very simple and intuitive to use.)

Part 5 looks at how food affects your body, for better and for worse, and presents a commonsense approach to eating for every goal.

Part 6 wraps it all up by celebrating the joys of lifelong lifting.

But first, I'll make this promise on behalf of Alwyn and myself: We will not claim to have invented anything that delivers magical results in minimal time. Resistance training itself has some magical properties—there'll be days when you feel like Superman just because you showed up and got a good workout in when you were tempted to blow it off. But we will not promise you anything that's outside the bounds of human physiology. Furthermore, we will not claim that we've invented workouts or techniques that do things other workouts and techniques can't do.

Sure, we'll take credit for explaining them in new ways, and Alwyn is one of the best trainers in the world when it comes to innovative program design. But there's a difference between explaining, popularizing, and synthesizing ideas—what we do—and creating new ideas out of the ether. We'll take great pains to give credit where it's due, but we'll also take credit for putting things together in a unique, interesting, and blessedly simple way.

Our goal here is to manipulate what is known about strength training so that it's as easy as possible for you to learn, as effective as it can be in the time you allot for it, and as enjoyable as anything else you would do with that time and energy.

That's right—this can and should be fun. It's fun to learn, it's fun to see the results, and it's fun to pursue for a lifetime. I was born in 1957, and I've been lifting since 1970. Granted, I didn't know what I was doing until I hit my midthirties. But it was always fun for me, even when I was clueless about what I was doing and why I was doing it. The more I learned, the more fun it became. I've probably enjoyed the past few years of lifting more than the decades that came before them. I've lifted heavier weights than ever before, with no injuries. How many people can say they're stronger and more muscular in middle age than they were in their youth, even when they spent that youth fit and healthy? I can, and by the time you're finished with this book, I think it'll be pretty clear that you can, too.

THE NOT-SO-FINE PRINT

Alwyn and I created this book to clear up the confusion about strength training, to sort out the many competing claims about different programs and training ideologies, and to make it simpler and easier to pursue for anyone who wants to pursue it.

We didn't write it for guys who have already spent successful, productive years in the weight room, or who are competitive athletes or aspiring bodybuilders or powerlifters. We like those guys just fine; our best friends and our most respected colleagues are all lifelong lifters, some of whom are accomplished athletes and guys who've won powerlifting and bodybuilding titles.

If those guys want to buy this book, that's great. We're 100 percent in favor of sales.

But we wrote it for guys who want to be lifelong lifters but struggle to become even monthlong lifters. We wrote it for guys who join a gym, get their two free personal-training sessions, and then wonder what the hell they're going to do next. We wrote it for the guy who shows up for his workouts, does what he thinks he's supposed to do, and asks why he's not getting the results he expected.

In other words, *The New Rules of Lifting* is a book for the guy who's been promised abs of steel but ended up feeling socked in the gut. It's for the guy who's gotten nothing from strength training beyond bulked-up B.S. and a slimmed-down wallet. We aren't promising abs like giant ravioli, slabs of pec meat, or biceps that have their own GPS coordinates.

Instead, we offer this:

- When you finish this book, you will know exactly what you're doing in a gym. You won't have to guess about the best exercises or workout systems. You'll know what perfect form looks like, and when you have it right.
- You'll also know what not to do. We'll steer you away from dangerous exercises, unproductive techniques, and self-sabotaging habits.
- You will discover why some lunatics like Alwyn and me consider exercise fun. You'll find that the knowledge you gain from *New Rules* will translate into results, results will translate into a better self-image, and a better self-image will transform exercise from a task on your "to-do" list to a pursuit you gladly build your days and weeks around.

TWO THINGS YOU WON'T FIND IN THIS BOOK

If you've read a few fitness and weight-loss books, you'll notice they typically include some elements that you won't find here. Such as:

Specific claims about the results you'll get in a finite period of time

Alwyn has created workouts for this book that I truly believe are better than any I've seen in print in my fourteen years as a journalist writing about exercise and fitness. But neither Alwyn nor I can tell you what kind of results you can expect or how fast you can expect them. We can't control your genetics, your diet, your effort, or whatever distractions interrupt your focus and separate you from your goals. All we can do is give you the best possible programs and the best possible instruction, and cheer you on. Actual results will vary.

Before-and-after pictures of people who've successfully used these workouts

Alwyn and I first started talking about working on a book together after he showed me pictures of one of his clients, a forty-year-old man who'd lost 100 pounds in a year of training with Alwyn. In the "after" picture, the man looked like he'd been lifting for his entire life—lean, muscular, strong. I trusted Alwyn because I know him, but anyone else would've had to study the two pictures for a while to figure out that it was the same guy.

We could've used those photos here as an illustration of the magic of Alwyn's workouts. And it would've been more honest than the supplement ads, with the pasty-skinned bodybuilders pushing their bellies out in the harshly lit "before" pictures and then pulling them in while covered with tanning cream and bathed in dramatic studio lighting in the "after" shots.

But we didn't. Alwyn's client made that transformation while being trained by Alwyn. This book comes as close to personal-training sessions as possible, but it's not the same thing. So we won't pretend it is.

CREDIT WHERE CREDIT IS DUE

Since Alwyn and I don't take credit for creating any of the ideas in this book, we'll give plenty of props to those who deserve it. But credit can sometimes overwhelm the idea that we're trying to get across. Take, for example, the following, which is only a slight exaggeration of the type of attribution you see in some fitness magazines:

> "Yes, that's right," says Hannah Rottweiler-Edelweis, Ph.D., R.D., P.T., M.I.C., K.E.Y, associate assistant professor of human binary eschatology at the Frances Fullington Beaningham Institution of Advanced Obfuscation at the University of Eastern South Dakota in Deadwood and author of *Humor in America: Why Laughter Could Be Good Medicine, Except When It's Not* (Conglomerate Press, 1997). "At least, I think it is."

To avoid all this, we'll have two designations for the experts whose ideas we cite: *, which means "bunch of letters after his name," or **, which means "tons of letters after her name."

* will describe experts who most likely have a master's degree, at least one major personal-training certification, and other professional designations, like R.D. or P.T. (registered dietitian, physical therapist).

Alwyn, for example, is a *: M.Sc. (a graduate degree in sports science from Chester College, University of Liverpool), CSCS (certified strength and conditioning specialist, awarded by the National Strength and Conditioning Association), MSS (master of sports sciences from the International Sports Sciences Association), CHEK (certified by exercise guru Paul Chek), USAW (certified to teach Olympic-style weight lifting), NASM–CPT (certified as a personal trainer by the National Academy of Sports Medicine), ACE–CPT (certified personal trainer by the American Council on Exercise), and ACSM–HFI (certified as a health and fitness instructor by the American College of Sports Medicine).

I don't really qualify as a *, since the only letters I have that matter are CSCS (My bachelor's degree is in journalism, making me one of the few who will admit he went to school for a B.J. But for obvious reasons, I don't put those letters after my name.)

** is for someone with a medical degree or doctorate, and then some of the stuff the * designees have. An example is my friend Susan M. Kleiner, Ph.D. (doctor of philosophy in nutrition and human performance), R.D. (registered dietitian), and FACN (fellow of the American College of Nutrition).

And at the end of the book, among the chapter notes, I'll tell you more about the studies and books from which we created these programs, and in some cases the *s and **s who conducted or wrote them. That'll give you a chance to look them up yourselves, to see if we merely borrowed or outright plagiarized the ideas contained in them.

Read on, and if all else fails, be skeptical.

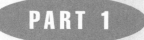

PART 1

FACTS

What Your Personal Trainer Forgot to Tell You

A GENERATION AGO, the idea that strength training was actually good for you—that it offered any health benefits, that it helped people live longer, that it did anything besides give you bigger muscles to flex or stronger muscles to push people around with—seemed absurd.

Kenneth Cooper** wrote this in *Aerobics,* his 1968 bestseller: "If it's muscles or a body beautiful, you'll get it from weight lifting or calisthenics, but not much more. . . . If it's the overall health of your body you're interested in, [strength training] won't do it for you. . . . Aerobic exercises are the only ones that will."

You may think, "Well, of course he'd say that. He had a book to sell."

And he sold a lot of books. He used some of the money to build the Cooper Institute for Aerobics Research in Dallas, the purpose of which was to promote . . . bodybuilding.

Sorry, just wanted to see if you were paying attention. Of course, the purpose of his center in Dallas was to encourage a type of endurance exercise he had dubbed "aerobics."

One study that came out of his center was published in 1992, and it offers proof that the anti-strength-training vibe was still going strong in academia well into the Arnold Era, when gyms were bulking up with free weights, and muscular icons like the Soloflex Guy and the *Men's Health* cover guy and even the Diet Coke guy flexed their way into the zeitgeist.

Researchers looked at the blood of thousands of men and women—heart patients at Cooper's clinic in Dallas—and also measured their muscular strength. They discovered that the strongest men had the highest triglyceride levels (which is bad) and also the lowest levels of HDL cholesterol (also bad, since HDL is the "good" cholesterol). Never mind that the people in the study, for the most part, weren't doing any strength training. The researchers still drew this conclusion: "These data suggest no beneficial effect, and perhaps an adverse association of muscular strength on lipid and lipoprotein status."

In other words, "Muscles kill!"

I'm not talking about an Internet posting here. The 1992 study appeared in *Medicine & Science in Sports & Exercise,* the most "official" of all exercise-science publications.

Since then, we've learned a lot about strength training and aerobic exercise. We now know that men who lift weights at least once a week for thirty minutes have 23 percent less heart disease than men who don't. (That's from the Harvard Alumni Health Study.) Cooper himself wrote a book called *The Strength Connection* in 1991, along with an anti-aging book in 1999, both of which advocated a mix of strength training and endurance exercise.

Other studies have shown that hitting the iron improves health in any number of ways. Cardiac rehab patients lift to help regain muscle mass. Diabetes patients pump iron so their bodies will better control their blood-sugar levels. (Bigger muscles give the excess blood sugar a place to go so it doesn't stay in the bloodstream and mess up the arteries.) Older adults work their muscles so they'll actually *have* muscles; research has shown that as little as two months of strength training can reverse twenty years of strength and muscle loss in seniors.

The rest of us just do it so we look good naked.

And there are a lot of us. According to American Sports Data, more than 39 million Americans now belong to health clubs. That's well over 10 percent of the adult population. More than 50 million trained with free weights, in some fashion, in 2003, and that's up 25 percent since 1998.

In a sense, my career—hell, my entire reason for being—has been vindicated. I started lifting in 1970, when I was thirteen. I'd never heard of Arnold Schwarzen-

Strength Kills? Hardly

At least four studies I know of have shown that the strongest men live the longest. Correlations to longer life have been found for grip, leg, and abdominal strength. This makes perfect sense, of course. We know that disability kills, and that strength is a powerful deterrent to the loss of physical mobility and function.

However, a 2004 study in the *Journal of Applied Physiology* found that muscle *power* is a better predictor of longevity than is muscle *strength*. Lots of studies have shown that power—the ability to generate force rapidly, such as a quick hop to avoid an obstacle—declines faster than strength does as we age. But this is the first study I know of that shows the decline in power directly affecting life span. This correlation held up even when the researchers adjusted for body size, muscle mass, and the amount of exercise and other physical activity of the participants.

Here's how it breaks down:

A fifty-five-year-old man who suffers the greatest decline in power, relative to other men his age, has just a 15-percent chance of living thirty more years. Someone with an average power decline has a chance of living to eighty-five that's just over 20 percent. But the men who lose the least power have a better-than-30-percent chance of living three more decades.

So the biggest spread occurs between the 50th and 95th percentiles; this is one case where it pays to be better than average. And the men who retain the most physical power have better than twice the survival rate of men who lose the most over the next thirty years.

Alwyn has made power exercises one of the most important components of his *New Rules* workouts—not to mention a unique one.

egger, and I never considered the health implications of what I was doing. All I knew was that I was skinny and weak, and lifting weights made me bigger and stronger.

That was good enough to keep me going for thirty-five years and counting, the last fourteen as a journalist writing about, and advocating, strength training. The rest—the health benefits and disease prevention—is just gravy.

The pro-muscle vibe is so intense in this country that I no longer have to explain to people why they should lift weights. Virtually everyone I talk to is already sold on the need to lift. But while I admire their enthusiasm, I often cringe at their methods.

See, I think a lot of people are wasting a lot of time and energy doing exercises, workouts, and routines that aren't particularly useful. When I see lifters hitting the gym three, four times a week and not getting bigger, leaner, or stronger, I wonder why they aren't changing their methods or at least investigating the possibility that there might be a better way to do what they're doing.

But before I get into that, I want to establish a few of my bedrock principles. These aren't the New Rules of Lifting; I self-mockingly call them Lou's Rules of Exercise. But I think they're worth stating, right up front:

LOU'S RULE #1 • Do something.

I'm as firm a believer in the benefits of strength exercise as you'll find. But I don't want to imply, in any way, that other types of exercises aren't beneficial. Exercise scientists don't agree on much, but I think they'd all acknowledge that the most important benefits of exercise accrue when someone goes from sedentary to moderately active. (And stays active—you don't get any points for your varsity letter if you're thirty-five and haven't exercised since high school.) Sure, there are greater benefits when you go from sort-of fit to really fit, however you choose to define "fit." But you get most of the good stuff just by getting off your ass and moving.

LOU'S RULE #2 • Do something you like.

I assume you're reading a book with the word "lifting" in the title because you like to lift and want to learn how to do it more effectively, or because you haven't lifted before and want to learn how to start off right. But on the off chance that you're reading this book because someone told you to eat your vegetables, and strength training is the New Spinach, I want to clear this up: You don't have to lift weights. It's not a rule. You won't build muscle and increase your strength if you avoid it. On the other hand, if you lift and do nothing else, you won't get all the benefits of other types of exercise, either. That's why Alwyn and I included the information about dynamic warm-ups, flexibility, and cardio exercise in Part 2. (Important fine print: When we use the word "cardio," we don't mean "aerobic" exercise. It's a fine distinction, but one Alwyn and I will explain carefully in Chapter 7.)

So my point here is that if you're following Lou's Rule #1 and doing something active, it's better to do something you like than something you don't. People who don't like the type of exercise they're doing will soon stop doing it. No one has the discipline to keep laboring in perpetuity at a non-income-producing activity they find unpleasant. It's why we have automatic dishwashers and lawn tractors.

Conversely, people who like what they're doing have a better chance of sticking with it.

I'm no fan of yoga or jogging, and I used to enjoy basketball until my knees finally demanded that I hang up my Air Jordans. (Which, if logos were honest, would've been called "Floor Schulers" when I wore them.) But I'm not going to talk you out of any type of exercise, as long as you enjoy it.

That said, bowling, skeet shooting, and playing golf in a cart barely count as exercise. If they're all that stand between you and the couch, okay. But I'm pretty sure you can do more than that.

LOU'S RULE #3 • The rest is just details.

Heretical as it sounds, my position as a fitness professional is that I want you to get up and move, and hope that you'll find something you enjoy so much that you don't resent having to get up and move.

Once you're moving and having fun, Alwyn and I could come up with a million ways for you to get better at it, to get more out of it, and to expand from it to other activities that offer different and important benefits. (Well, Alwyn could come up with millions. I could come up with hundreds. Or dozens. At least five or six . . .)

But those are the details. You'll get almost all the real improvements from following Lou's Rules #1 and #2.

Enough with the windup. Here's the pitch.

FIRST, ROUND UP ALL THE TRAINERS

Walk into any gym in America, and you'll see some strange stuff.

You'll see guys who're fifty pounds overweight doing set after set of biceps curls, as if the ego-boosting effects of having seventeen-inch biceps will somehow negate the metabolic damage inflicted by a forty-six-inch waist.

You'll see skinny guys working their chest muscles through dozens of sets of redundant exercises, without even glancing over at the squat rack, which is the one place in the gym where they're almost guaranteed to pack on the muscular weight they want.

You'll see a guy with flab hanging over his belt crunching and crunching and crunching some more, in hopes that a low-intensity exercise involving very little muscle mass will somehow magically melt off fat that, thanks to a fluke of human physiology, just happens to be adjacent to those small working muscles.

You'll see young guys lifting way too much weight with bad form, older guys lifting way too little weight on machines that require almost no attention to form, and everyone plodding along on treadmills and recumbent bikes with little idea of why they're doing it. (In fact, one of the oldest jokes in the gym is about the guy who'll circle the parking lot for fifteen minutes to get the space closest to the front door, then go in and walk on the treadmill for a half hour.)

As you go through *The New Rules of Lifting,* you'll learn why each of the things described above is ill-advised at best. But here's a quick preview. If you take away nothing else from this book, I hope you'll remember these rules of productive strength training.

NEW RULE #1 ● The best muscle-building exercises are the ones that use your muscles the way they're designed to work.

During the millions of years in which the human species was evolving, our bodies developed to accomplish certain basic tasks: running, jumping, climbing; throwing, hitting, and twisting to dodge throws and hits; pushing things away, pulling them closer; lifting things off the ground, throwing things down to the ground; squatting down, lunging forward.

We can still create hundreds of exercises based on those actions, but we can also eliminate an even greater number of exercises that have nothing to do with basic human movement.

NEW RULE #2 ● Exercises that use lots of muscles in coordinated action are better than those that force muscles to work in isolation.

Isolation exercises have their place, and some trainers use them successfully when teaching their clients the basics of strength training. But most of the time, the average person in a health club gets little benefit from a biceps curl, lateral raise, or leg extension. Harking back to New Rule #1, those muscles weren't designed to work in isolation, so exercising them that way is almost always a poor use of your valuable time and energy.

This is one of those rules that seems intuitively wrong to most people. If you want bigger biceps, why wouldn't you do biceps curls?

I'll explain that in much greater detail later in this chapter, but for now I'll leave it at this: If you were being chased by a lion across the savanna and your only hope for escape was to pull yourself up on a tree branch, would you try to curl yourself up onto that branch, using your biceps in isolation? No, you'd grab that branch with both hands and pull with every damned muscle in your body that could save you from becoming the leonine equivalent of a high-protein lunch. (Lions are the original Atkins dieters.)

No matter how big and strong your biceps are, they're of little use to you unless all your other pulling and climbing muscles are proportionately strong.

I know you don't go into the gym thinking, "What can I do today to save myself from a future lion attack?" But here's why the lion matters: Your body has no reason to develop your biceps so that they grow out of proportion to other muscles on your body. That would make you biomechanically dysfunctional, and your body will resist that.

Besides, once you start isolating all the little muscles on your body, you commit yourself to spending a lot more time in the gym. (And, no matter how much you like them, biceps really are puny compared to the muscles of your chest, back, and thighs. Mine are, anyway.) But even if you have all the time in the world, Alwyn and I hope to convince you that you'll be better off doing more basic, streamlined workouts.

NEW RULE #3 ● To build size, you must build strength.

Big muscles are metabolically expensive. It takes a lot of energy and effort to build and preserve them. Your body will resist building those big, costly muscles unless it perceives a good reason to do so. That reason is strength. If your muscles need to get bigger to accomplish specific tasks, they'll grow (assuming you give them enough food).

And make no mistake: Muscle growth through increased strength is *always* your goal in the gym. You aren't in there to "tone" your muscles, which implies that you're just adding a bit more tension to your muscles than they have now. You could do that in a yoga class.

All the good things you want from strength training come from building bigger, stronger, more powerful muscles. Those muscles will help you control your weight (via metabolic processes that I'll explain in Chapter 7). They'll provide protection against injuries. They'll roll back the aging process, giving you a body that performs as well as one twenty years younger. (Alas, they won't prevent shoulder hair, but they could help you hook up with someone who'll shave it off for you.)

The Perfect Man, the Perfect Workout

At the turn of the century, a strongman and bodybuilder named Eugen Sandow became one of the most famous people in the English-speaking world. Even today, a likeness of his muscular physique—he stood about five-foot-eight, weighed 180 pounds, and had a twenty-nine-inch waist—is used on the trophy given to the winner of the Mr. Olympia contest.

The irony is that bodybuilding contests represent the opposite of what Sandow did to build his famous muscles, and what he promoted.

You can see his workouts for yourself on a variety of websites. I went to sandowplus.co.uk and downloaded a chapter from *Sandow's System of Physical Training,* published in 1894. Most of the "heavy-weight exercises" he recommends for advanced athletes involve lifting a weight overhead, with the weight often starting on the floor. He claims to have been able to perform a one-arm snatch—a continuous motion, lifting a dumbbell from floor to overhead—with 186 pounds. But that pales compared to his best-ever "one-handed slow press from the shoulder": If his own book can be trusted, he once pressed 322 pounds with his right arm. (His record for his left arm was a mere 300.)

It's hard to imagine one of today's 300-pound bodybuilders even trying to shoulder-press that much weight, unless he was sitting on a bench with his back fully braced, and using both hands. And yet Sandow, at 180 pounds, standing on the floor, could do it with one hand . . . and no steroids.

NEW RULE #4 • To build size and strength, you must train hard but less frequently, with plenty of recovery time between workouts.

I don't want to scare you off with the "hard" part. I mean it in a relative way: To get the full effects of strength training, it's better to train harder and less frequently than to take it easy on yourself but work out more often. Again, this seems to go against popular wisdom and perhaps even common sense.

Why wouldn't more exercise be better? Because, to be effective, muscle-building exercise must inflict some damage within your muscles. I'm not talking about the kind of damage you'd suffer in a car accident. You don't need to cripple yourself to put a little meat on your bones. (Although, believe me, many have tried.)

Saved by the Cough

In May 2004, I tried to join a local gym in Allentown, Pennsylvania. My wife was a member, and she'd always raved about the place. The gym's head trainer, John Graham,* is very active and well known in the National Strength and Conditioning Association, of which I'm a member and from which I'm certified as a strength and conditioning specialist.

In other words, it's my kind of place.

While I was filling out the paperwork to join, a trainer nervously asked me my age. "Forty-seven," I answered, with some pride. I may not look like a guy who writes weight-lifting books for a living, but I'm in damned good shape for a middle-aged man who sits at a desk most of the day.

"Um, before you can work out here, you need a doctor to sign a release."

"A release? Me?" I showed him my NSCA credentials.

"Sorry, it's a rule. If you're over forty-five . . ."

The irony here isn't just that I'm a fitness professional being told I need a doctor—any doctor—to give me permission to exercise at their gym. Just two days later, I received a National Magazine Award for an article called "Death by Exercise." (It was part of a winning package of three stories entered by *Men's Health* in the Personal Service category.) The article described how and why people die while exercising, and anyone who read it carefully would know that someone could pass a pre-exercise checkup with flying colors and go out and drop dead on the track an hour later.

Since I'd never be caught dead on a treadmill, the chance of me dying in their gym was pretty close to zero. Almost all deaths attributed to strength training involve accidents, and most of them occur at home. A guy will try to bench-press his maximum, fail to get the weight up off his chest, and watch it roll up onto his trachea.

Still, I did go to see a doctor, and the checkup ended up being useful. He looked at my throat, saw it was irritated from my seasonal allergies, and suggested a nasal spray that helped me breathe easier.

But enough about my nose. My goal here is to tell you that, if you're really overweight, really out of shape, and really over forty, you should get a checkup before you work out.

One more personal story: I once helped put together a training program for an overweight relative. Almost as an afterthought, I suggested he see a doctor first. He did, and found out he had a hernia. He got surgery, and began the program when his doctor gave him clearance.

Moral of the story: When in doubt, see a doc. You never know. . . .

But you do need to put in enough effort to create some sort of disruption within your muscular structures, usually including some mild inflammation. And then you have to leave the weights alone long enough to allow your body to repair those tears. The result: bigger, stronger, more injury-proof muscles.

Now let's go to the next chapter, to see how you'll go about tearing those muscles down.

Introducing the Big Six

I'M GOING TO MAKE a horrible confession about my own ignorance. When I conceived this book, I had a brilliant premise: I would take every exercise in the gym and look at it in terms of its possible role in human movement. The only good exercises would be those that mimicked important hominid actions—jumping, running, pushing, pulling.

I wanted my list to come down to just five or six movements, and then build the entire book from there. So, convinced of my genius in being the first to come up with this idea, I worked on it for weeks.

Finally, I e-mailed Alwyn with my list and my idea that the most useful movements also build the most muscle mass.

Alwyn wrote back a short e-mail (I think the man is incapable of being long-winded), saying, "Well, in that case we should go with squat, bend (deadlift), lunge, push, pull, twist. That's according to Schmidt's theory of human movement." In a later, equally short e-mail, Alwyn mentioned the seventh movement, walking or running, which doesn't necessarily have to be trained with gym exercises, provided you're doing some of that outside the gym. (And if you're not . . . why aren't you?)

So this Schmidt guy (known to his admirers as Richard A. Schmidt**) had stolen my idea and, worse, stolen it at least three decades before it occurred to me. What's more, Paul Chek,* an exercise maverick, had already used Schmidt's theory in articles and books, and he'd come up with a list of basic movements that was almost identical to mine. (Check out the page 288 of the notes section for a more detailed explanation.)

Now let's step out of the confessional and take a look at the six key movements.

✳ Squat

WHAT IT IS: In the gym, the most common version you'll see is the one with the barbell across a guy's shoulders. You can also do the exercise with dumbbells held down at arm's length, although that version's a bit awkward, since you have to hold the dumbbells slightly out to your sides to keep them from bumping into your knees. If you're using challenging weights, you end up using your upper-body muscles a bit more than you want.

MUSCLES USED: The great thing about the squat is that it uses virtually all the muscles in your lower body in one movement. The biggest challenge is to your

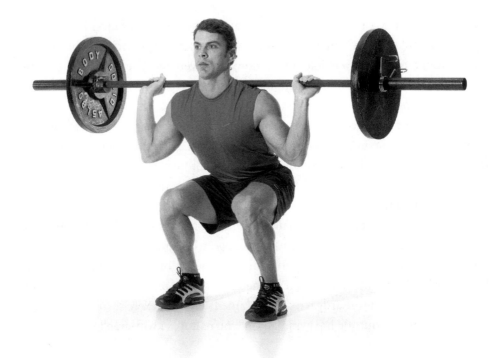

quadriceps, the muscles on the fronts of your thighs. These muscles are responsible for straightening your knees when they're bent. (There are some caveats to this muscle-use explanation, which you'll find in Chapter 8.)

But the exercise also works the big, powerful muscles surrounding your hip joints. These include your gluteals (buttocks) and hamstrings (rear thighs). The lower you go on the squat, the more these muscles engage.

Your lower-back muscles also play a role, mostly to keep your torso upright while you're squatting down and straightening back up. Many muscles help keep your body stabilized, from your feet to your calves to those in your inner and outer thighs, on up to your abdominals and middle back.

REAL-LIFE USES: Strength coaches know that if they want to increase an athlete's jumping ability, the squat is the most important exercise. It's not the only exercise, of course, but the fact that it's been shown in many studies to increase vertical-jump height shows how important the squat is to a very basic human movement.

So how important is jumping? After all, most of us don't jump at all once we get past our jockstrap days in high school and college.

Imagine a ninety-year-old you. It's 2065, and you're sitting in a chair in front of the TV. It's a comfy chair, and you think you could spend the rest of your days sitting there, watching 125-year-old Alex Trebek wheezing questions to centenarians on *Geriatric Jeopardy*. ("Senior moments for five hundred, Alex." "Eh?" "What?" "Sorry, the answer is 'Metamucil.' Pick again.")

Suddenly, nature calls. You try to get up. Nature calls again, louder this time. You try again to get up, but your atrophied lower-body muscles just can't summon the strength and power to get you out of that chair. Nature gets tired of calling, and just shows up. In your lap.

I know you aren't going to hit the gym today to avoid soaking your favorite chair sixty years from now, just as I know you don't go through life worrying about lion attacks. But you don't just wake up one morning without the ability to get up from a comfy chair. There's a slope—with age, you gradually lose strength and power until you have trouble walking up stairs, playing with your grandkids on the floor, and, yes, getting out of bed or a chair.

✳ **Deadlift**

WHAT IT IS: You bend over a barbell or pair of dumbbells and lift it or them off the floor by straightening your body at the hips.

MUSCLES USED: Like the squat, the deadlift and its many variations use just about all your lower-body muscles, but this time the emphasis is on the powerful gluteal and hamstring muscles that straighten your hips.

Your lower back has an important role in stabilizing your body while bending and straightening, along with your deep abdominal muscles. Your trapezius—the big, diamond-shaped muscle that runs from your neck to your shoulder blades to your middle back—also has a big role in this exercise, since your shoulder blades have to pull together in your back to finish the movement. Finally, the gripping muscles in your hands and forearms get a workout, since without a strong grip that barbell is going to slip from your hands and hit the floor (if you manage to lift it off the floor at all).

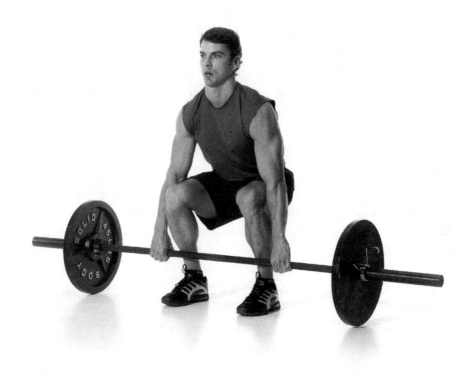

REAL-LIFE USES: It's hard to go through life without picking heavy stuff up off the ground, which makes the deadlift perhaps the most useful exercise you can do with weights.

Imagine a life in which you couldn't lift a sleeping child off the floor, or move a sofa, or pick up a box of books without one of your spinal discs turning into sushi. (A friend of mine who had back surgery tells me the stuff that spills out of a ruptured disc looks like crab meat. Just FYI.) You wouldn't want that life. The deadlift and its many variations keep your back and hips strong.

✴ Lunge

WHAT IT IS: You hold weights at your sides or across your shoulders (or do it without weights), take a long step forward, and descend until your rear knee nearly touches the ground. Then you push off with your front leg and step back to the starting position.

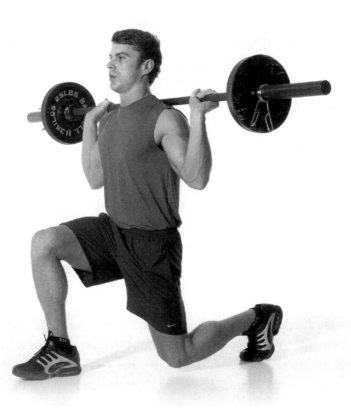

An alternative is the "split squat," in which you start the exercise with one leg already out in front, and then lower yourself and rise again without stepping out and back.

A third variation is the "step-up," in which you step forward and up onto a platform.

MUSCLES USED: This exercise uses the same muscles as the squat and deadlift, but in a crucially different way. On the front of your pelvis are muscles called "hip flexors," which lift your thighs up in front of your torso. (The opposite muscles are the "hip extensors," the gluteals and hamstrings, which straighten your torso when it's bent forward.)

Most people have tight hip flexors—a lifetime of sitting will do that—and in some they're so tight as to be locked up, practically. The tighter your hip flexors, the harder it is to jump, much less take those long steps forward or diagonally to get over a puddle or avoid a snoozing drunk on the sidewalk.

The lunge forces those muscles to stretch and then contract quickly. That makes it one of those exercises that's as much about increasing the suppleness and flexibility of your muscles as it is about keeping them strong.

REAL-LIFE USES: Almost all sports, excluding chess, feature lunges to the front or side. Imagine a baseball infielder who couldn't lunge to stop a grounder up the middle, or a beach volleyball player who couldn't lunge to dig an opponent's shot out of the sand.

The lunge also figures into those powerful strides a sprinter takes to get up to full speed, and the move a wrestler uses to take down an opponent, and the step you take before throwing a ball. And what is soccer but a series of lunges in every direction?

I understand you probably aren't playing any of these sports right now. But the lunge is still crucial to your everyday physical well-being. The shorter your strides, the less mobile and agile you become. And when mobility and agility go, you're just one slip or tumble away from the assisted-living community, where you sit back in that comfy chair to watch TV . . .

✳ Push

WHAT IT IS: It can take many forms in the weight room, such as a push-up, bench press, shoulder press, or dip. In a push-up, obviously, you push your torso up from the floor. In a bench press, you lie on a bench, lower weights to your chest, then push them back to arm's length. An overhead press involves pushing the weights straight up from your shoulders. A dip starts with your bent arms behind you (your body is "dipped" down below them), and is completed by straightening your arms and pushing your body up even with them.

MUSCLES USED: Even though the push-up and bench press are generally thought of as "chest" exercises, and the overhead press is a "shoulder" exercise, and the dip is a "triceps" exercise, they all start with action in your shoulder joints. The dip, push-up, and bench press mostly activate the front parts of your shoulder muscles, while the overhead press uses the front and middle parts.

The push-up, bench press, and dip use your chest muscles in conjunction with your front shoulders. The overhead press bypasses the chest muscles and instead uses more of the shoulder muscles.

All four exercises use your triceps to straighten your arms at the elbow joint.

REAL-LIFE USES: Many in the gym would consider the two major pushing exercises—overhead press and bench press—to be physiologically distinct. Certainly, you wouldn't do one and expect to get all the benefits of the other. But outside the gym, the line blurs. You're rarely pushing straight off your chest (a chest pass in basketball is one of the few exceptions I can think of) or straight overhead. Most movements are at an angle in between the two extremes.

Imagine this: Your neighbor's car has slipped off the road on a snowy day. You get behind the car to push it back onto the road. How's your body positioned? Chances are, your torso is at a 45-degree angle to the ground. So, although most of your power is going to come from your legs, you're still going to use your chest, shoulders, and triceps to push. That's not a pure analog of any gym exercise. In fact, while it might start off resembling an incline bench press, it quickly morphs into more of a shoulder press as you push the car farther from your torso, and as your torso lowers to a position that's almost parallel to the ground.

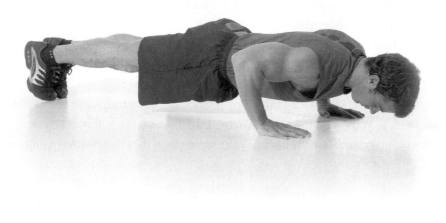

Let me take that a step further: If Alwyn and I could design a gym, with no limits on space or expense, we'd probably have a lot set up just for pushing cars around. We couldn't invent a greater exercise for developing total-body strength and muscle mass, assuming we could find a way to rig it so the cars would move in a straight line with no chance of rolling back over an exhausted pusher. Beginners would push stripped-down Mini-Coopers and Toyota Tercels, while advanced guys would shove armor-plated Lincoln Navigators. (Admit it: You'd love to work out in that gym.)

Pushing moves also figure prominently in sports. Most throws are types of pushes, since they finish with you straightening your elbows. For example, a football pass is a combination of a lunge-step forward, a push, and a twist (discussed below). Punches are also push-twist combinations, and the traditional bully's shove is a pure push.

And, although the last thing I want to do here is write a sex book, you can't ignore the fact that the same muscles you use in a push-up are the ones that keep you from crushing your beloved (or at least beliked, however briefly and transiently) in the missionary position.

✳ Pull

WHAT IT IS: As with pushing movements, pulls can come from many angles. The lat pulldown—one of the most popular gym exercises—involves pulling a weight straight down to your shoulders from overhead. In a pull-up or chin-up, you pull your body up to a stationary bar.

Rowing exercises have many forms. In a gym, you can sit at a machine and pull a weight toward you. You can also sit or stand in front of a cable pulley and pull a weight toward you from many different angles, using one arm or two.

Free-weight rowing exercises are usually done with you bent over at the hips so your torso is nearly parallel to the floor. Then you pull dumbbells up to your sides, or a barbell up to your abdomen.

Finally, there's the pullover, in which you take a weight that's overhead or behind you (if you're lying down) and pull it in an arcing motion until it's in front of or over your torso.

MUSCLES USED: The two major upper-back muscle groups are the latissimus dorsi—"lats" to you—and the trapezius, or "traps." The lats are shoulder-joint muscles; they pull your upper arms back to your torso when they're extended overhead or

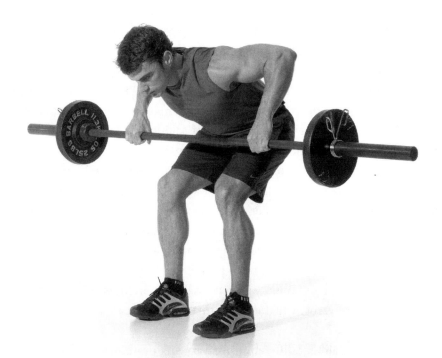

in front of you. The traps are shoulder-blade muscles, meaning they pull your shoulder blades together in back (as in a row), or down (as in a pulldown or pull-up), or up (as in a shrugging motion).

Your biceps and some of the muscles in your forearms aid your lats (and, indirectly, your traps) in these pulling exercises. That's one of the most important points we'll make in this book: Your biceps will get all the work they need from rows, chin-ups, and other pulling exercises. They don't really need any special attention to grow in proportion to the rest of your muscles. And, as I've already said in this chapter, they won't grow out of proportion to those muscles no matter how many curls you do, and no matter how you do them.

I won't make the argument that curls don't do anything—any time you work a muscle directly, it'll get bigger and stronger. And if you want to give them direct work, I won't talk you out of it. Alwyn's workouts include a few biceps curls, strategically inserted at various points in the training scheme. I'll even confess that, when the weather warms up and the long-sleeve shirts go to the back of the closet, I'll throw some curls into my workouts. But my big point remains: Over the course of your lifting life, your biceps will do just fine without any special attention. They'll get bigger and stronger if the rest of your muscles get bigger and stronger. And they won't change shape no matter what you do—that's all determined by your genetics.

REAL-LIFE USES: If I could design any exercise machine, it would be one that mimics a tug-of-war. I don't think there's another exercise or game that so thoroughly works your biceps and upper-back muscles in their natural, harmonious relationship to each other. (With the possible exception of sailing in a heavy wind; I'm not the nautical type, so I have to take the sailors' word for it.)

If you're winning the tug-of-war, you're starting the pull with your upper-back muscles, then finishing with your biceps and, to a lesser extent, your forearm and hand muscles. (Don't underestimate the importance of grip strength—it's one of the few aspects of muscular fitness that's been linked to a longer life.)

In fact, if you put together all the components of a successful tug, you'd start with a straightening at the hips that resembles part of the deadlift motion, then a pull with the upper back, then a biceps curl, with a twist thrown in for good measure. In other words, in one picnic game, you'd employ three of the six most important muscle-building movements.

Tug-of-war isn't all that different from a rowing movement, and of course rowing is called "rowing" because it mimics the very useful act of (ready for this?) rowing a boat.

The other important use of the pulling muscles is in climbing, an ability that was so important to our primitive ancestors that it literally meant life or death. If you couldn't pull yourself up into that tree or scramble up that cliff faster than whatever drooling predator was in pursuit, you were that day's low-carb lunch special. And there goes your genetic legacy—a tangle of bones and a few steaming piles of saber-tooth-tiger dung in the Pleistocene forest.

In climbing, you start to pull yourself up using your upper-back muscles, then finish with your biceps. And, of course, you can't get around the importance of gripping strength. You slip, you die.

One more point about pulling movements: They mirror pushing movements precisely. For example, if you were tugging on a rope with one arm, it would be the mirror opposite of a pushing motion. In the gym, the shoulder press and pull-up are opposites, as are rowing and bench-press movements. You could even do the opposite of a pullover, if you wanted to do an exercise called a "front raise," in which you lift a weight in an arcing movement from the front of your torso to overhead.

With muscles so clearly designed to mirror one another, it's crucial to give them equal emphasis in the gym. You won't have to worry about muscle-use discrepancies if you follow Alwyn's workouts, which are perfectly balanced. But when you're on your own, you'll probably revert to the common gym ratio of three to one—three times the time and effort on the front-body muscles as the ones in your back. And you'll probably do a lot of curls, too, which won't help the situation. You'll soon end up with overworked, overtight muscles in the front part of your shoulder joints, putting too much strain on the comparatively weak muscles in the back of your shoulders.

Curls Gone Wild!

Part of my living derives from my ability to answer questions from readers. It's a growth industry—there's never a shortage of questions to answer. One of the classic questions: "My elbow (or wrist, or forearm) hurts when I do curls. How can I make it/them stop hurting?"

The answer is pretty easy: Stop doing curls!

But the problems encountered by my correspondents pale compared to this one, detailed in the March 2004 issue of *The Physician and Sportsmedicine.* The article was a case report of an eighteen-year-old football player who'd developed a condition called bilateral musculocutaneous nerve palsy from doing too many biceps curls.

The player was sent to his team physician after he tried to flex his biceps in the mirror and discovered he had no biceps to flex. That is, he couldn't get them to contract. The nerves controlling biceps action had shut down. This was after his biceps had gotten progressively weaker in the previous three weeks of workouts.

The cure? Stop doing curls! In three months, he was fine.

✳ Twist

WHAT IT IS: Some exercises are specifically designed to isolate the twisting motion. You can do this lying flat on your back and then twisting at the waist to lower your legs to the floor. Or you can anchor your lower body, and turn your shoulders from side to side, as in the Russian twist.

But you can also add twists to other gym exercises. For example, a standing row can include a twist, as can a shoulder press.

Finally, an exercise doesn't have to involve an actual twist to work the twisting muscles. If you do an exercise that requires coordination and balance, and you're actively *preventing* your torso from twisting, you're still using those muscles. That's why, when you get to the workout section, you won't see a twisting movement in every single program. Rest assured, though, that Alwyn took this movement into consideration and made sure it was covered, one way or another.

MUSCLES USED: Your waist has two sets of muscles charged with bending and twisting: the external and internal obliques. The internals lie beneath the externals, and the two sets of muscles have fibers that run diagonally in opposite directions. If you were to bend to your left, then straighten, the internal and external obliques on the right side of your torso would stretch as you bent and then contract to lift you back up. If you were to twist to your left, you'd use the external obliques on your right side and the internal obliques on your left side.

Some small lower-back muscles also play roles in bending and twisting. (The

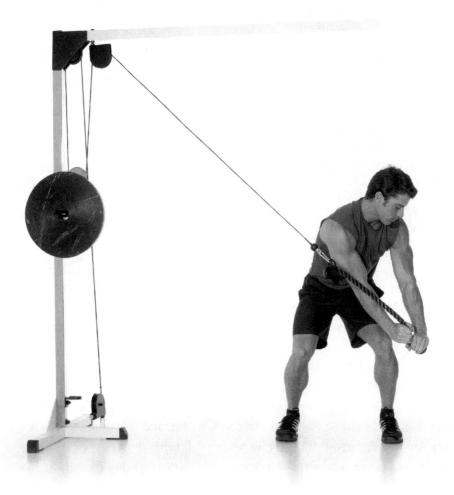

main lower-back muscle group, the spinal erectors, is mostly involved in straightening your back when it's bent forward.)

And, of course, the muscle you probably care most about, the rectus abdominis or six-pack muscle, is also involved in twisting. But its relationship to functional waist movement is so complex and, yes, twisted that I'd rather leave it out here so I can discuss it in appropriate detail in Chapter 13.

REAL-LIFE USES: You can't play a sport without twisting. The most obvious example is the baseball swing. A right-handed hitter will swing using the external obliques on the right side of his body, and the internal obliques on his left, to drive the ball, although most of his power will come from his hips as he turns them. (Many youngsters mistakenly believe that the forearms are the key to the swing, but the hands and lower arms are just the end of the whip. The hip turn is the key.)

Many trainers and gurus, such as the aforementioned Paul Chek, write and speak extensively about the importance of the midsection muscles as the communications link between your upper- and lower-body muscles. And Alwyn and I certainly don't disagree in general (although we might quibble with some particulars of each trainer's approach—we fitness geeks are good at quibbling).

But the importance of abdominal strength, flexibility, and overall integrity goes far beyond sports. Your day starts with a twist, when you throw your legs over the side of the bed to walk to the bathroom. (And if you don't start the day by going to the bathroom, you're probably not drinking enough water. But that's a subject for Chapter 22.)

From there, nearly everything you do involves a series of bends and twists, separately and together. You twist getting in and out of your car. You twist in your chair at work to get a file. You bend and twist to pick up your kids, or pick up after them.

You've probably heard that 80 percent of Americans develop back problems at some point. It's one of those statistics I've used so many times that I couldn't tell you where it started, or whether it's still true or ever was true. But even if it's the scientific version of an urban legend, it's worth repeating just to get people to pay attention to the importance of midsection fitness. Strong abdominal muscles may not prevent back injuries—most guys train their abs with series of crunches, which aren't thought to do much, if anything, to protect your spine. But midsection fitness does. That includes endurance, strength, and flexibility in all your mid-body muscles, which Alwyn's workouts will promote.

✳ **Walking and Running**

WHAT THEY ARE: As I said earlier, you rarely need to train these movements in the gym. In fact, the idea of running with weights in a gym seems like a major injury or accident begging to happen. You may as well pull out your cell phone and dial 9 and 1 before you even start.

However, you can build good exercises around walking. One is called the farmer's walk, a staple of the Strongman competitions you see on ESPN. You hold heavy weights in your hands and walk a specified distance, sometimes with steps to climb up and down. Another, promoted by trainer Chad Waterbury, is a figure-eight movement, in which you hold a barbell overhead with straight arms while walking in intersecting loops.

MUSCLES USED: Your entire lower body gets involved in walking and running—in fact, walking and running are pretty much the main reasons you *have* a lower body. Your hip flexors (muscles on the front of your pelvis) lift one leg up and out in front of you, while your hip extensors (gluteals and hamstrings) and calves on your trailing leg push against the ground to propel your body forward. The muscle on the front of your shin, the tibialis anterior, lifts your toes up on your front leg so they don't drag on the ground.

Meanwhile, your postural muscles, such as your internal obliques and some of the small, strut-like muscles in your lower back and hips, keep your body upright and stable while you move.

You'll notice that I haven't mentioned the quadriceps, the big muscles on the fronts of your thighs. Their main job is to straighten your knees when they're bent, and that's not hard to do while walking or running. Runners are notorious for having tight hips and hamstrings and relatively weak quadriceps, while lifters sometimes are the opposite—they do so many leg presses and leg extensions for their quadriceps (the muscles they can see in a mirror) that they end up with relatively weak hamstrings. Either combination is bad for your posture and the health of your knees and spine.

REAL-LIFE USES: I don't need to belabor the importance of walking or running, since they're part of everything. I will, though, mention that running *fast* is one of the great neglected exercises in our world, even among those who are fit.

As with jumping, few of us have a need to approximate a sprint as we get older. And when we try it, it tends to be at a company picnic or some other occasion in which we go from zero—no warm-up, no momentum—to full speed in an instant.

Changing the Bodybuilding World, One Phrase at a Time

One phrase you won't see in *New Rules* is "body part." (Or, as the bodybuilding magazines say, "bodypart," as if making it one word somehow legitimizes it.) Bodybuilders love to talk about their routines for this body part or that bodypart (depending on their choice of reading material), as if their bodies were simply collections of muscles that could be assembled and shaped any way they choose.

Quick story: When I was fitness editor at a magazine, a junior editor there, a nice young guy who clearly wanted my job, told me one day about his front-shoulder routine. He had three different exercises that he did for the front part of his shoulder muscles, and he thought I could use the routine in the magazine.

I don't remember exactly how the conversation went, but I remember thinking how bizarre it was to do three separate exercises for a single muscle that's about the size of two fingers. That muscle gets worked pretty hard already in pushing exercises, so it's hard to imagine a universe of fitness-magazine readers who were truly underdeveloped there, relative to the rest of the muscles surrounding their shoulder joints.

But after I left and he succeeded me as fitness editor, sure enough, he ran his shoulder routine—three exercises for a muscle that hardly anyone needs to exercise in isolation in the first place.

To me, that's body-partism run amok. Bodybuilders develop entire routines for muscles like biceps and rear shoulders, which should get plenty of work from the basic exercises in their workouts. Certainly, bodybuilders are different from the rest of us—they're training for an aesthetic ideal and are willing to devote nearly unlimited time and energy to that pursuit. And the final product, if it works, is a physique in which all the "body parts" are in proportion to one another.

Of course, there are some problems with that approach. For one thing, when you teach your muscles to work in isolation, you run the risk that they'll forget how to work together. That's why you rarely see high-level athletes with bodybuilder physiques. And the ones who develop them often become more famous for their pose-worthy muscles than for their athletic accomplishments.

It's not that you can't develop a fantastic-looking physique while also training your body to work in harmony in sports competition. It's just that bodybuilding-type workouts accomplish the former while hindering the latter. If you get your six-pack abs and peaked biceps because you've taught those muscles to work and grow in isolation, you've developed the look of an athlete while diminishing your ability to actually perform like one.

That's why Alwyn and I advocate a different way to look at your physique in general and your training in particular. If you focus on integrated movements, rather than exercises chosen for their ability to isolate "body parts," you'll build the same muscles but end up with a body that actually knows how to use them, as opposed to a body that just knows how to pose them.

Granted, that full speed won't be very fast, but it'll be very tough on muscles that aren't used to it. Once I pulled a quadriceps muscle doing exactly that in the first softball practice of the season—with no warm-up, I tried to chase down a fly ball, and I pulled the muscle on the first or second step. I could just as easily have pulled a hamstring or calf. (I tore a calf muscle one time playing basketball, but that wasn't from being ill-prepared so much as playing on a cold night on a concrete court, and playing against an idiot who decided to throw the ball against my lower leg as hard as he could so it would go out of bounds.)

So, while running fast is great, starting off slowly makes it even better.

The Building Blocks of Muscle

You may have guessed, in reading Chapter 2 as carefully as you did, that there's more to muscle-building exercise than knowing six basic movements. And you're right. Even if you know the six movements, and dozens of exercises based on those movements, you still have no idea how to work out.

At this point in the book, I could simply hand you off to Alwyn, and you could do his workouts for the next year, and you'd get great results. But that would be too easy. (Not to mention perplexing to my editors, who thought I was going to write a book, as opposed to retyping a series of workouts.)

I think it's just as important to understand the goals of training, rather than just the methods. The methods are interesting—I've been writing about them for fourteen years, and I haven't gotten bored yet—but they have a lot more meaning when you know why they exist.

I'll tell you about the concrete stuff—sets, repetitions, weights—in a moment. First, though, ponder these:

NEW RULE #5 • The goal of each workout is to set a record.

By the end of every workout, you should have accomplished something you haven't done before. That doesn't mean a maximum lift—you won't worry about that for a long time. It's much broader than that.

It could mean a higher volume of exercise—more combined lifts than you did the last time you performed the same workout.

It could mean that you did the exact same volume as the last workout, but with heavier weights in some lifts.

But it will probably mean a combination of those two parameters—on some exercises, you used more weight for the same total of lifts, and on others you did more total lifts with the same weight you used last time. And on still other exercises, you were lucky to duplicate what you did last time, because you pushed yourself to beat your personal records on other exercises.

The big rule is this: Never do the exact same workout two times in a row. You always want an improvement in something.

NEW RULE #6 • The weight you lift is a tool to reach your goals.
It is not a goal by itself.

Weight lifting and powerlifting are terrific sports. So are Strongman competitions, the Highland Games, and other organized contests that involve feats of maximum strength and strength endurance.

But those are sports—exhibitions of the results of hard exercise. They are not exercise in themselves. When you walk into your workout space with the purpose of exercising, your goal is to improve some parameter of your function and physical appearance.

So, before you begin these workouts, forget any ideas you had about how much you want to bench-press. Forget any preconception about the size of the dumbbells someone of your magnificence should be able to work out with. You will work out with the weights that allow you to accomplish the goals of your workouts, no more and no less.

If you use too much weight, you can't complete the workout as designed. If you use too little, you can complete the workout *without achieving the goals* of the workout.

However, if you're going to err—and all of us have to use trial and error to pick the right weights when we're doing new exercises or routines—it's best to take your risks on the light side, and then use heavier barbells or dumbbells in subsequent sets or workouts. Don't fear light weights because you think someone might laugh at you. Speaking as someone who's seen his share of dummies with dumbbells, the guys using too-heavy weights always look more ridiculous than the ones using too little.

That said, if you're intimidated by the heavy iron, I want those thoughts stopped, too. You may very well be capable of using more weight than you've used in the past.

NEW RULE #7 ● Don't "do the machines."

I've had this conversation so many times I've lost track. A man or woman says to me, "I'm not getting anything out of my workouts." I ask what they're doing. He or she will say, "I do the machines."

"The machines" is a reference to the circuit of devices designed to work all the muscles in isolated safety. In a basic gym, you might find . . .

- four leg machines (leg extension, leg curl, leg press, calf raise)
- three pushing machines (shoulder press, chest press, triceps pushdown)
- four pulling machines (lat pulldown, some kind of horizontal row, pullover, biceps curl)
- two middle-body machines (some kind of crunch for your abdominals, some kind of back extension for your lower back and gluteals)

You might also find a machine for twisting at the waist, along with a "pec deck" for working your chest and a lateral-raise machine for your shoulders.

Notice what's missing from this list: None of these machines comes within spitting distance of mimicking the squat. (The leg press is thought to, but doesn't; see "Exercises We Hate #1" on page 32.) The leg extension and leg curl condition muscles, but they don't imitate any movements that are actually useful in real life. (Not an issue with bodybuilders, of course, but a big problem for everyone else.)

Only one movement—the back extension—imitates the deadlift. And we like the back extension, as long as you do it on the device known as a Roman chair, as opposed to the weight-stack machine, which is dangerous. (See "Exercises We Hate #2" on page 33.) But it's not the same as picking up a weight off the floor.

None comes close to the lunge.

The pulling exercises aren't horrible. In fact, they're the best, most useful machines in the gym, and they're the only machines that actually improve on what you

Bad Press

The exercise: 45-degree leg press

How it works: You load up the leg-press apparatus with hundreds of pounds of weights, then set your-self in the machine with your back against a pad and your feet on a platform. You push the platform until your legs are straight, then lower it again. Ideally, you start and end each repetition with your knees bent 90 degrees. In reality, many lifters go deeper, which causes their hips to come up off the pad, rounding the lower back.

Why we hate it:

1. It's a completely nonfunctional movement. It's hard to think of a real-life action in which your back is anchored and you push out with your feet to move a heavy object.

2. It's sneakily dangerous. Once your hips come off the pad, you're putting your lower back in jeopardy, according to Stuart McGill** in his book *Low Back Disorders.*

3. It's too damned easy. Bodybuilders love this exercise because they can load up the machine with half the plates in the gym (it's not unusual, in a hard-core gym, to see guys leg-pressing more than 1,000 pounds for reps). But if any of these guys could squat even half of that, I'd be surprised. So you get the worst of several worlds: You get to lift a whole lot of weight without actually accomplishing anything.

4. Most guys will hold their breath as they're lowering the weights, which, given the fact your legs are coming up toward your chest, almost certainly means you're creating an off-the-charts surge in blood pressure.

What to do instead: A squat offers all the benefits but a fraction of the dangers. If, because of pre-existing lower-back problems, you can't do squats safely, McGill recommends doing leg presses with just one leg, leaving the other foot on the floor. That will keep your back from coming off the pad. But McGill adds this: "We still consider this a nonfunctional motor/motion pattern."

can do with free weights, to a point. (You'll find lots of pulling and twisting exercises in Alwyn's workouts that use cable machines.)

But the pushing moves are a disaster. Shoulder-press and chest-press machines don't allow your shoulders to choose their own range of motion. Even worse, they're built with the premise that both your shoulders have the exact same mechanics. The odds that they do are about zero—one shoulder is usually a little wider than the other, if not torqued or twisted so it's higher, lower, forward, or behind the other. Pushing a fixed bar through a fixed range of motion is ridiculously risky for most lifters.

Then there's that crunch machine or, more accurately, the trunk-curl machine.

EXERCISES WE HATE #2

Disc Hole Inferno

The exercise: machine back extension

How it works: You strap yourself into the machine, bend forward so your spine is rounded, then push backward against a pad until your back is arched.

Why we hate it: The machine exerts a compressing force on your spinal discs while you're extending backward. In *Low Back Disorders,* McGill describes the exercise as "the easiest way to ensure herniation" of a disc. A few sets probably won't do any damage, but the heavier the load you use, the fewer sets and reps it takes to make a disc go boom.

What to do instead: McGill's studies have shown that the key to lower-back health is muscular endurance, not strength or flexibility. So if you have a healthy back, and do the exercises Alwyn has chosen for *New Rules,* you'll develop endurance. That's because exercises requiring balance and coordination force the small, strut-like muscles in your lower back to work hard to keep you upright.

Would you believe me if I told you that this movement is worthless? Of all your abdominal muscles, the one targeted by the crunch—the rectus abdominis, better known as the six-pack—is functionally the least important. It has almost no role in protecting your spine, although it is involved in integrated actions with the other abdominal muscles in sports and other dynamic movements. And I'll concede that no abdominal exercise truly isolates one set of muscles, so even a crunch works more than your six-pack. But if you try to justify the crunch in terms of human function, it's hard to make a case. Your body has hardly any need to bend forward at the waist while your lower body is anchored. (There are exceptions. If you combine the crunch with another type of movement, such as throwing a ball, or a balancing component, it becomes a much more interesting and useful exercise. Alwyn has a few you'll enjoy trying.)

Again, our case against machines will proceed throughout *New Rules* on a case-by-case basis. For now, I want to emphasize two points.

1. Many machines force your joints into unnatural ranges of motion, creating damage that may take years of treatment to repair.

2. Most machines prevent your body from doing the most important and useful muscle-building movements.

NEW RULE #8 • A workout is only as good as the adaptations it produces.

This is similar to New Rule #5. You want to set a record during each workout so that you force your body to make adaptations that will lead to greater strength and muscle growth. At a certain point—and that point will be a moving target throughout your lifting life—your body won't be able to make adaptations to your current workout. That's when it's time to move on to the next workout.

Alwyn's *New Rules* programs are designed with the idea that you'll make adaptations to each workout in four to eight weeks. The older and more experienced you are, the faster you adapt. Conversely, the younger and less experienced you are, the longer you can stick with one program and still get benefits.

But there's a bigger philosophical issue here, beyond the matter of how often to change exercises around. Those guys who tell me they "do the machines" and then wonder why they aren't getting results? Most have been doing the exact same routine, in the exact same way, as long as they've been lifting. Many will tell me they've been using the same weights most of the time.

Sometimes I want to weep for guys who confess they've been doing the same routine for three years when they should've switched after three weeks. Well, not really. I don't feel sympathy so much as I want to throttle whoever should've told them to make changes but didn't bother.

THE UNSALTED NUTS AND BOLTS OF LIFTING

Let's assume you remember some elementary science and know that your body is made of atoms, atoms form molecules, molecules combine to form compounds, and those compounds somehow come together to form interesting pieces of flesh like blood, skin, and hair (among those lucky enough to have any). Put together those pieces of flesh in the right way, and you have an organism.

Repetitions—individual lifts—are the atoms of strength training.

Sets—combinations of repetitions—are the molecules.

Exercises are compounds—that is, they're performed in sets of repetitions, and you can change the sets and reps around any number of ways to produce different compounds.

Workouts are collections of exercises you decide to put together and perform in one session. At this point, you have something that you'd recognize as part of an organism.

That organism is your **program**.

Just as your liver or rib cage is pretty worthless outside the context of your fully functioning body, so a workout is just a curiosity when you consider it in isolation. Alwyn could write the greatest program ever put into an Excel spreadsheet—and even I could write a decent one—but if you don't use it within the context of a program, it's of little use to you.

Let's take a closer look at each component.

REPETITIONS

If a repetition is the atom of a muscle-building program, then the separate parts of a repetition are its subatomic particles. The part you think of as a "lift" is only one of three components of a repetition. The others are the lowering of the weight and whatever pause you take between lifting and lowering.

The lifting portion has two formal, scientific names: You can call it the **_concentric_** or **_positive_** part of the repetition. (Or you can just call it "the lift." I'm easy.) What you're doing here is forcing your targeted muscles to contract. The purpose of any action of your skeletal muscles is to work joints, which moves bones closer together or farther apart (or keeps them from moving closer together or farther apart, as explained below).

Of course, when you lift weights, the last thing you're thinking about is what your bones are doing. But I think it's important to remember that your body is in the bone-moving business. Muscles only grow in proportion to their strength, and their strength is their ability to move heavy objects with those bones. That heavy dumbbell in your right hand is an impediment to the movement of the bones in your arms. Thus, the muscles controlling your elbow and shoulder joints must get stronger. And, most of the time, that extra strength will lead to more size.

Your muscles also have to work during the lowering part of a repetition, which has two scientific names: **_eccentric_** or **_negative_**. You can probably guess that your muscles are better at lowering heavy weights—that is, controlling the descent of those weights—than they are at lifting. A guy who would strain to bench-press 200 pounds for a single repetition could easily control the descent of a 240-pound barbell down to his chest, and do it multiple times. (Assuming he has strong people there to help him lift it off again.) But you probably don't know that the negative portion of a repetition has been shown in some studies to produce more muscle growth and strength improvement than the positive.

Some advanced training programs feature "negatives"—repetitions designed to force your muscles to lower extremely heavy weights—and in my experience they certainly help increase strength and size. But trust me when I say that negative reps beat the hell out of your muscles and joints, and you have no business doing them until you've tried everything else and built a considerable base of strength and muscle size.

Finally, there's the pause, which in some contexts can also be called an *isometric* contraction. Most lifts have two pauses: at the bottom, after you've lowered the weight to the starting position; and at the top, after you've lifted it and are about to start lowering.

You can manipulate the pause for different effects. For example, let's say you're doing a chin-up. You pull yourself up to the bar. The easiest thing would be to lower your tired self immediately. But if you pause in that position, holding your muscles in an isometric contraction, you've just made the exercise a lot more difficult. I recently did a program in which I did sets that started with a single chin-up, held at the top position for twenty seconds, followed by however many normal chin-ups I could do. To say those sets reduced me to a quivering, whimpering sack of once-proud manhood would be mostly accurate. But I think my arms grew a quarter-inch that week, so the temporary loss of pride was worth it. Still, I won't pretend I felt that way while I was still twitching uncontrollably.

The pause at the other end of a repetition—after you've lowered your body or the weight—has a different purpose. It won't build muscle and strength, but the longer you hold that pause, the harder the next repetition will be. That's because you've neutralized the natural elasticity of your muscles, their ability to snap back from a stretched position to a flexed position.

You can try it in your next workout: On one set of each exercise, pause with the weight in a lowered position for a count of five, then do the repetition. It'll feel different, I guarantee. You'll have to work with lighter weights, or do fewer repetitions, or both.

SETS

This is a group of repetitions that you perform one after another, usually without a break. If you're really curious and spend a lot of time searching for new and different workout systems, you'll find that sets can include one repetition or a hundred, and many configurations in between.

But, most of the time, sets will look like this:

Twelve to fifteen repetitions

This is best for developing muscular endurance and learning the feeling of muscular exhaustion. Don't laugh; lots of people have no idea what it feels like to have muscles so tired they won't do another repetition, no matter how hard you beg. You can experience some muscle growth with high-rep sets like these, especially when you're a beginner. But if you continue doing high-rep sets after the first few weeks of lifting, you'll prevent muscle growth. Don't laugh at that, either; Alwyn and I could run out of fingers and toes counting the number of people we've met who were afraid of getting "too bulky," and thus did high-rep sets to the exclusion of exercise that might actually be useful to them.

Eight to twelve repetitions

This is the classic bodybuilding configuration, meaning that over time these medium-duration sets have become the gold standard for muscle-focused workouts. And it's easy to see why. Way back in 1945, an Army physician named Thomas DeLorme used strength training to help soldiers recover from injuries and wounds. Eventually, through trial and error, he came up with the most famous strength-training protocol ever: three sets of ten repetitions per exercise, otherwise known as 3 × 10.

DeLorme also came up with the idea of a strength-endurance continuum that's been mostly unchallenged in the sixty years since. He believed that heavy-weight, low-repetition training produced the best strength gains, while moderate-weight, medium-repetition work (i.e., 3 × 10) produced the best gains in muscle size. And light-weight, high-rep sets induced improvements in muscular endurance without doing much to boost strength and size.

I'll quibble with some of that in a moment. But for now, let's say DeLorme was mostly right, and that medium-rep, medium-weight training is at least one of the best protocols for inducing the mechanical stimulus needed to gain muscular size.

When I say "mechanical," I mean the physical act of moving bones from one spot to another with heavy objects attached. But there's more to building muscle than simple mechanics. Your hormones play a significant role, and multiple studies by William Kraemer** show that medium-rep, medium-weight sets with short rest periods in between are best for stimulating growth hormone and as good as anything else for getting your testosterone into action.

Growth hormone and testosterone are your body's most important muscle-building hormones, and growth hormone also stimulates the fat-burning process. So you have a lot of things going right, physiologically, when you crank out sets of eight to twelve reps with little rest in between. You have a good mechanical stimulus for muscle gain, you have your hormones cooperating to build muscle and burn fat, and you're also working with weights that your body can handle with little risk of injury.

Three to six repetitions

Many still believe that DeLorme got it right back in 1945: Heavy weights and low reps will increase strength, but to increase muscle mass you need to do more repetitions with lighter weights.

I, too, used to believe that, until I shifted to heavy weights and lower repetitions in my own training. That's when I made what may be the most important discovery of my thirty-five years of training: I could build much more muscle, and build it much faster, with heavy weights and low reps.

A 2002 study in the *European Journal of Exercise Physiology* backs me up (kind of): It shows that, when novice lifters were put on low-rep, heavy-weight programs, they gained at least as much muscle as novice lifters on medium-rep, medium-weight programs, and quite a bit more than the beginners doing high reps with plastic Barbie weights.

I think the fact that someone as experienced as I am made sudden gains on low-rep, heavy-weight programs shows two things:

1. The longer you lift, the heavier you have to go to see gains.
2. You'll almost always see results when you do something you haven't done before.

There's also a pretty good testosterone response to low-rep training, which should help build bigger muscles. Another benefit: If you're doing a technically complex lift, something that takes a lot of practice, it makes more sense to do low-rep sets, since your form will start to break down as you get into higher reps. But I'm getting ahead of myself.

EXERCISES

The research I mentioned above regarding testosterone and growth hormone showed a link between specific exercises and hormonal response. Exercises like squats, which use the body's biggest muscles, produce the best possible hormonal response.

I used a lot of black ink in the first chapter explaining why some types of exercises are better than others, so I won't belabor this here. Simply put: chin-ups, good; biceps curls, mediocre. If you're flying blind in the gym and working without a written program, you'll always do yourself a favor by expending the most energy on the exercises that use the most muscle.

That said, there's a lot more to exercise selection than merely choosing the "best" exercises and assigning them a system of sets and reps. I think you can accurately divide exercises into these two categories:

Structural exercises

The Big Six—squat, deadlift, lunge, push, pull, twist—are structural. That is, they involve coordinated movements that your body needs to be able to perform.

Assistance exercises

These movements help you get better at the structural exercises. Let's say you do an upper-body workout that includes four structural exercises: chest presses, rows, shoulder presses, and chin-ups or lat pulldowns. (I know I don't get any points for creativity here.) After doing those four, you might finish up with lateral raises to strengthen your shoulders, along with some arm exercises. Or you might do pullovers to work your chest, upper back, and triceps from a different direction.

Sometimes the structural exercises themselves become assistance exercises. Let's say you're doing heavy bench presses, and follow that with push-ups with your hands on a ball or balance board. Now you're using a structural movement—the push-up—to develop coordination and shoulder stability, along with strength in the mid- and lower-body muscles that have to work hard to keep you from losing your balance and doing a face-plant on the floor.

The key: You can build an entire workout around structural movements, but you can't—or shouldn't—build one around assistance exercises. And yet about three-quarters of the bodybuilding playbook is assistance exercises. I've said it before and I'll say it again: That's fine for them. But you deserve better.

WORKOUTS

Just to make it simple, I'll say there are two main types of workouts:

Total-body workouts

To most people who've been lifting for a while, this seems impossible: "How could I possibly do three or four sets of eight to twelve reps of all thirty-seven exercises in my workout plan?"

And there's no way to answer that, except to ask, "Why are you doing thirty-seven exercises?"

Of course, the reason is pretty obvious. The bodybuilding magazines have made strength training so complicated that every guy thinks he needs to do at least six exercises for his biceps and triceps alone. That's not counting the three he does for his calves; the three he does for his front, middle, and rear shoulders; and the half-dozen or so he does on the floor for abs. That's eighteen exercises right there, before he does a single squat, deadlift, bench press, or pull-up.

And the women in the gym haven't escaped the workout-inflation cycle, either. Equipment manufacturers have convinced them they need to do special exercises to open and close their legs, and the stomp-aerobics cartel gave them another set of moves for their buttocks.

So the only people who actually do total-body workouts are the poor saps doing "the machines," mindlessly pushing and pulling on weights that wouldn't challenge a prepubescent spelling-bee champion.

Alwyn and I happen to be fans of total-body programs. If you simply do our Big Six for two or three sets each, you have a perfect workout with just six exercises to remember.

You don't sacrifice any benefits for that simplicity. You still work all your body's muscles, major and minor, and work them hard. You get all the hormonal benefits of strength training, since those come from the big-muscle exercises. It's the best of all worlds—no muscles missed, no time wasted.

However, at a certain point, most of us will find that it's hard to put equal effort into six structural exercises in a single workout. Maybe we start with squats and deadlifts, and then we're too wiped out for the pushes and pulls. Or, for no reason but vanity (which is fine; I consider vanity highly overrated, as deadly sins go), we work ourselves into pumped-up splendor on the upper-body exercises and have nothing left for the squats and deadlifts.

At that point, it's time to explore . . .

Split routines

I could think of dozens of ways to split up workouts, and Alwyn could come up with dozens of variations on every program on my list. And we'd still miss a few.

The idea is simple: By spreading your structural exercises over two or three workouts (or, in the case of bodybuilders, five to twelve), you make sure you have enough energy to work as hard as possible on each of them. Then, by finishing each workout with assistance exercises, you ensure that you improve your strength, muscle mass, and structural integrity with each workout—and you probably recover a little faster, too, since you aren't completely wiping yourself out every time you step into the weight room.

A few classic splits:

UPPER-BODY/LOWER-BODY I think every lifter, at some point, gravitates toward this one. Most of us will start our workout week with the upper-body workout (specifically, with bench presses; I think 95 percent of all lifters on earth do their bench presses on Monday). This will include at least two types of pushes (chest and shoulder presses), two types of pulls (rows and pulldowns, or pull-ups), and then whatever goofy arm, shoulder, and ab exercises we delude ourselves into thinking will make us more buff and lustworthy.

Enlightened lifters will then focus on squats, deadlifts, and some strategic assistance exercises in the lower-body workout. Typical lifters will avoid those exercises, since they require coordination and effort, and will instead go for leg presses, leg extensions, leg curls, and calf raises. We can only weep for them, and hope they someday see the light.

PUSH/PULL The idea here is that you work your "pushing" muscles (chest, shoulders, triceps, quadriceps, calves) in one workout, and your "pulling" muscles (upper back, middle back, lower back, gluteals, hamstrings, trapezius, biceps) in another.

This type of routine seems out of vogue these days, but twenty-five years ago, I can remember lots of guys doing them. I think the modern equivalents of this are the various bodybuilding splits described below:

THREE-DAY SPLIT Experienced lifters who want to hit it hard three times a week often move toward this configuration, and there are countless ways to do it. Most typical, I think, is the upper-lower-upper split. That is, you do upper-body exercises on Monday and Friday, and lower-body moves on Wednesday.

For instance:

MONDAY: bench presses, rows, bench-press variations (incline, decline, close-grip), row variations (cable, dumbbell, wide- or underhand-grip)

WEDNESDAY: squats, deadlifts, lunges, and some variations on those

FRIDAY: chin-ups or pull-ups (or lat pulldowns), shoulder presses or upright rows, dips, and perhaps some arm exercises (although if you do chin-ups and dips, your arms have already gotten a pretty thorough workout)

FOUR-DAY SPLIT My favorite four-day configuration is one Ian King uses in his more advanced workouts, which you can find on t-nation.com. I use his terminology to describe them:

"Horizontal push/pull": These exercises include bench-press and row variations.

"Hip-dominant": Here, he means deadlifts and deadlift-type exercises—anything that starts with action from the powerful gluteal and hamstring muscles.

"Vertical push/pull": These include pull-ups and pulldowns, as well as shoulder presses and upright rows, plus dips and pullovers.

"Quad-dominant": You could also say "knee-dominant," since these are the exercises that are more dependent on the muscles surrounding the knee joint. So squats are the featured exercise here, but he also includes leg curls, which bodybuilders would include with their deadlift variations.

WESTSIDE SPLIT Louie Simmons and the powerlifters at Westside Barbell in Columbus, Ohio, use this four-day split:

"Max-effort squat": This routine involves one heavy lower-body move, a variation on either the squat or deadlift, followed by assistance exercises for the lower body.

"Max-effort bench": Same thing, except the max-effort exercise is a bench-press variation, and it's followed by assistance exercises for your upper body.

"Dynamic-effort squat": The goal here is to develop movement-specific speed and power in the muscles used in the squat and deadlift.

"**Dynamic-effort bench**": Same thing, but with the goal of developing more speed and power in the bench press

BODYBUILDING SPLIT The idea is to isolate muscle groups ("bodyparts") and work them to exhaustion, as if they were revolutionary insurgents in a third-world country who had to be divided and conquered. I've seen bodybuilding routines with twelve workouts a week—two a day for six days. Entire workouts might be devoted to biceps or triceps or hamstrings, isolating these muscles from the ones they're designed to work with. If Alwyn and I believed in this type of training, we'd show you how to do it. But we don't, so we won't.

PROGRAMS

If you take away nothing else from this chapter (and I'll concede, it's a damned long and exhausting chapter), I want you to remember this: The best trainer in the world could write the best workout in the world, but unless it's in the context of a good program, it does you little good.

Let's run through a hypothetical situation: On January 1, our trainer hands you this workout. On January 2, you rush to the gym and try it. You hit it hard, and come out sweaty and tired and sore and happy, and think, "Damn! That was a great workout!"

So what do you do the next time you're in the gym, on January 4? Same thing? How about January 6? How about the workout after that?

Your body will adapt to that workout sooner or later, and if you don't have something else to do, something that moves your training forward and builds on the adaptations the workout produced, you're not much better off than you were before the world's best trainer handed you the world's best workout.

But let's say, on January 1, you were given the gift of the perfect workout after reading this book. Since you memorized all twenty New Rules, you know that, according to Rule #5, your goal in the gym is to set a new record each workout. So now you're modifying the workout as you go. You're either working with heavier weights on each exercise or doing more sets and/or reps.

That's terrific. But how long do you think you can keep setting those records? You're going to get to a point at which you stall. If you're a beginner, you may be able to keep making gains for eight to twelve weeks. If you're advanced, you may not be able to go for longer than two weeks before you max out.

At that point, you can make one of these adjustments:

Increase weights, drop reps, take longer rest periods between sets

This will extend the life of a workout by weeks, if not months. Let's say most of the exercises in the workout start out with DeLorme's 3 × 10 configuration of sets and reps.

After four weeks, say, you decide to change it to 4 × 8, using heavier weights. That makes your workout longer and harder, and certainly would produce some new adaptations. You'll get stronger, you'll build more muscle, and with the increased volume and effort, I'd bet on you getting leaner, too.

Three weeks later you go to 5 × 5, and you get stronger and bigger and possibly leaner, too, although my guess is that you're eating a lot more at this point (heavy weights make me hungry as hell). So maybe you're getting *a lot* bigger and stronger, but your waist is also thickening a bit.

After three weeks, you go to 8 × 3, and do that for another three weeks.

Now you've taken that single workout and made it last thirteen weeks. You've gotten tremendously stronger, and you've put on some serious muscle, but possibly some fat, too. Worse than the extra fat, your joints are aching and you're bored out of your skull from doing the same exercises over and over for three months. So what else can you do?

Decrease weights, add reps, and/or decrease rest periods between sets

Now you're going for a different type of adaptation. You're working faster, sweating more, and creating a metabolic disruption that will cause some fat to melt off. (My colleague Craig Ballantyne* has a fat-burning program he calls Turbulence Training, for this reason.) You're also, most likely, generating a considerable growth-hormone response to your program, and that's going to help your body use even more fat for energy.

Let's say you can do that for three weeks before you're absolutely sick of working yourself into a clammy-skinned froth every time in the gym. You'd pay the world's greatest trainer a year's wages to give you a new workout. In fact, you're so burned out that you take two full weeks off from training. Then, at the end of the second week of loafing (wasting time by helping your kids with their homework, volunteering at the animal shelter, or distributing blankets to the poor—anything to keep you out of the gym), you hit on a new way to tweak your workout.

Change the exercises

Instead of doing flat bench presses, you do them on an incline, and maybe you switch from a barbell to dumbbells.

Now, charged up by the fact you get to do new exercises (and feeling refreshed after two weeks away from the weights), you start the workout over again, and progress through all the configurations: 3 × 10, 4 × 8, 5 × 5, 8 × 3, Turbulence. Let's say you do each for two weeks this time, and take two more weeks off at the end, because training that hard still kicks your ass, as it should.

So let's review:

Weeks 1–13: Worked with progressively heavier weights, increased sets, decreased repetitions. You steadily increased your strength and muscle mass but probably added some body fat, particularly in the later weeks.

Weeks 14–16: Switched to an intense, metabolism-disrupting, growth-hormone-generating, fat-melting program.

Weeks 17–18: Took time off for rest, recovery, and making the world a better place.

Weeks 19–28: Went through the cycle again, this time with different exercises.

Weeks 29–30: Took two more weeks off to save your body and improve the lives of those less fortunate than you.

You get back from vacation, and you're ready for new challenges in the gym. So you pick up your workout again, and you write out new exercises for yourself to do. But before you go to the gym with your new exercises and run through all the configurations again, you think about what you've liked and haven't liked about your previous months of workouts.

By this point, you've gotten to know your body pretty well, and you know that on certain exercises, you just don't seem to get much benefit from lifting really heavy weights with low reps. And, on others, the higher-rep sets don't seem to offer much benefit. You can't, for example, think of any reason to do three sets of ten deadlifts, or even 4 × 8. You know your form would slip anytime you got past the fifth repetition, so you think, "I should start deadlifts with 5 × 5."

Then you think about some other exercises you do, and realize that you can think of lots of better ways to do them. Sometimes, on assistance exercises, it's clear to you that you can get all the benefits of the exercise with a single, all-out set. On others, you do better with more sets but fewer reps.

So you organize all the exercises you like and seem to benefit from. You add the exercises you've always wanted to try but haven't fit into your program. You take the most important exercises, the structural ones, and put them first in your workout. Then you put the assistance exercises after them. And you configure the sets and reps according to how important the exercise is to you and how much benefit you think you get from it.

Then you realize that you have too many exercises and sets to do in a single workout, so you create a split routine, and decide you're going to do more sets, with fewer weights and heavier weights, of the structural exercises at the beginning of each workout. And you're going to do more reps, with fewer sets and lighter weights, of the assistance exercises.

Furthermore, you realize that you'd really like to improve your strength, and so you decide you're going to go all the way down to single-rep sets on the squat, deadlift, and bench press. You give yourself until the end of the year to do this, and you devise a way to change your workout every three weeks so you can gradually increase the weights and decrease the reps on your key structural exercises.

Now you not only have a split workout, you have a split workout that changes every three weeks to help you get the adaptations you want.

Fast-forward to January 2 of the following year. You run into your hypothetical best trainer in the world, and he looks at you and says, "Holy shizzle! Look at you! You've gained at least twenty pounds of muscle, and your waist is smaller!"

You tell him you've actually gained twenty-one pounds of muscle, put three-quarters of an inch on your arms, and lost two inches off your waist. You feel better than you ever have in your life, and just a few weeks earlier, you set personal records in the bench press, squat, and deadlift.

"I knew I was brilliant," the trainer says. "In fact, the whole world knows that, since my mom posted it on the Internet. My first three wives left me because they said they couldn't possibly rise to my level of perfection. But even I didn't know I could write a single workout that would transform a sorry schlub like you into the halfway-decent-looking person standing before me and basking in my reflected glory."

Then the trainer looks down at the workout sheets you printed out and carry on a clipboard. "What's that?"

"That's your workout." You see the look of confusion on his face. "Oh, I changed a few things," you add. "Like the sets. And reps. And exercises. And I made split routines. And I change them every three weeks so I can keep making adaptations. Other than that, it's exactly what you gave me a year ago."

"Of course it is!" the trainer agrees. Then he makes photocopies of all your workout sheets and uses them to train the rest of his clients.

But of course, it's not his at all. You've taken a single workout and transformed it into a genuine program, based on your abilities, your goals, and your strengths and weaknesses.

In other words, you've taken a rib cage, and from it you've created a living, breathing organism.

And you've also proved that you're smarter than the world's greatest trainer.

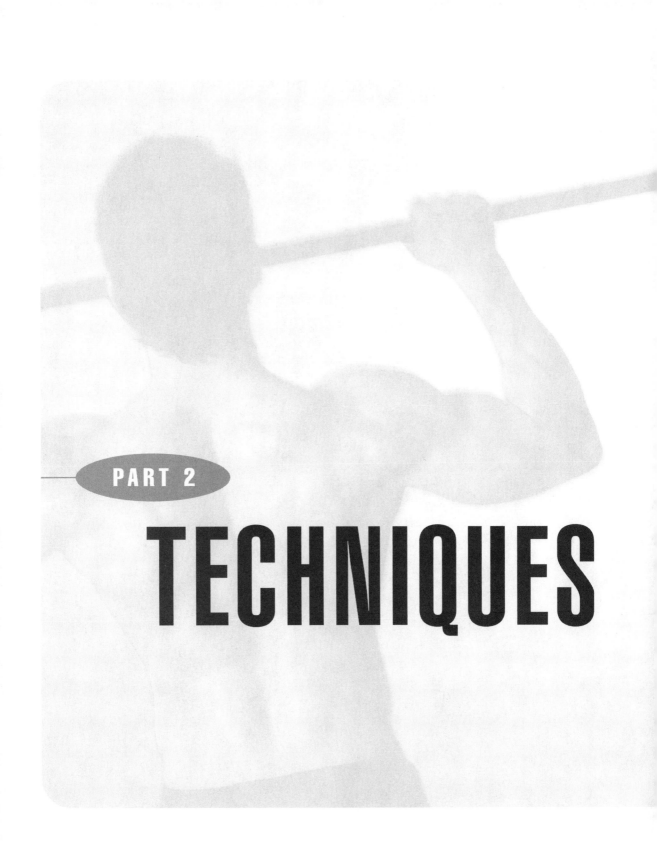

PART 2

TECHNIQUES

The Best Muscle-Building System for Almost Everybody

Take a deep breath. Get out of your chair. Walk around. Do a few lunges and twists to loosen up the joints in your hips and lower back. Feel better? Good.

That was a lot of information in Chapter 3, and I appreciate the fact you read it all the way through. In fact, you could stop reading now, jump straight to the workouts, and understand all the basic ideas that Alwyn used to create his programs.

But if that's all I told you, I'd feel I hadn't given you your money's worth. Sure, you could launch into the workouts without reading these next two chapters, and do fine . . . for a while. But it would be like cutting off your antibiotics the first day your throat stopped being sore. You haven't killed the bacteria; you're just giving them a chance to regroup.

Here's what I mean: You do Alwyn's workouts for eight weeks, maybe ten, then one day you pick up a bodybuilding magazine and see a new workout. And you think, "Hey! Look at all those curls! That would be a hell of a lot more fun than what I'm doing now. Plus, this shiny 290-pound guy who's too short to ride the Screaming Eagle at Six Flags says it'll add an inch to my arms!"

In this chapter, I'm going to explain the permanent way out of the darkness. It's a

51

concept of program structure called "periodization." Yes, it's a big word, and it doesn't exactly trip off the tongue. But the concept is easy to grasp, and it's crucial to understanding what it takes to build the body you want in the time you have.

First, though, allow me to serve up a few more rules.

NEW RULE #9 • There is no magic system of exercises, sets, and reps.

You could go through hundreds of legitimate studies of strength training, and you'd find any number of systems that work. At least, they work for somebody, and they work for a while. Every good and honest trainer knows these two corollaries to New Rule #9:

- Everything works.
- Nothing works forever.

That's why guys who advocate extreme systems, like Super Slow or High-Intensity Training, can claim that they've found the keys to the kingdom, and if you just do it their way, you'll be the coolest tool in the pool.

But I'll let you in on a little secret: Most of the guys who tell you about the magical system they've discovered, and have big ol' honkin' muscles to show for it, *built those muscles doing something else.* They'll tell you, with a straight face, that the methods they used to build their biceps and pectorals were crude and inefficient, if not flat-out dangerous. They were lucky to build those muscles without their arms falling off and their kneecaps exploding like ligamentous hand grenades. Yet, mysteriously, they offer no tangible proof that the new, enlightened system works even half as well as the techniques they now say are crap.

And even if you do find someone who clearly has a better physique with the Enlightened Way than he had back when he lifted in darkness, how could you ever prove he wouldn't have built at least as good a physique using other methods?

You can't, and that brings me to the next rule:

NEW RULE #10 • Don't judge a system by the physique of the person promoting it.

Even if you could find someone with a great build and prove that he indeed had more success with the system he now promotes than with any other, you still don't know anything useful about that system. All you know is that it worked for him.

As a fitness professional, I can't tell you how depressing it is when someone judges your knowledge by the size of your arms. Granted, I'd have my doubts about a fitness expert who clearly wasn't in shape, since there's both an art and a science to training. You'd hope the guy designing your program or dispensing advice genuinely loves to lift, and knows from his own experience how exercises are supposed to feel.

But in a universe in which most of the practitioners are in at least decent shape, it's pointless to pick the guy who's in the *best* shape and decide he must be the most knowledgeable. It may mean he has the best genetics, or the most discipline, or the most time and energy. But it absolutely does not mean he knows more than the guy with smaller arms or a weaker bench press.

This is yet another way in which modern bodybuilding has polluted the conversation about fitness in general, and about strength training in particular. The original twentieth-century bodybuilders were strength and power *athletes.* Take John Grimek, one of the real legends of the bodybuilding world: The man not only had the best physique of the 1940s, he was one of the strongest men of his time. He competed on the U.S. Olympic weight-lifting team in 1936, and at one time he held the American and world records for the military press.

He wasn't a natural for Olympic lifting—he was much better at slower lifts—but his strength is astounding at any speed. Here's an anecdote, recorded in John Fair's *Muscletown USA*: In 1940, in an exhibition in San Francisco, Grimek was challenged by a local strongman, a Norwegian fisherman. The local picked up a 240-pound barbell from the floor with a palms-up grip, curled it to his shoulders, then pressed it overhead. (Nifty thing to know: The reverse-grip shoulder press is called a "continental press.")

Despite the fact he'd never lifted weights that heavy with that grip, Grimek matched him. The contest ended when Grimek curled and continental-pressed 280; the Norwegian tried it but failed.

Grimek was a normal-size man: five-foot-nine, probably between 180 and 185 pounds. (At about that same time, he competed in weight-lifting contests at 181 pounds.)

I don't want to violate New Rule #10 and pretend anyone can look like Grimek or gain that kind of strength by doing his routine. The man may very well have had the best genetic combination for strength, muscle mass, and low body fat in the history of the world.

I just want to make the point that he wasn't a bodybuilder in the modern sense— he didn't spend hours in the gym strapped into muscle-isolating machines (they didn't even exist back then) or make sure he was sitting down with his back braced before he attempted heavy shoulder presses. He lifted the way everyone lifted back then—floor to ceiling. The weights usually started on the floor, and they often ended up overhead.

And yet he managed to become the best-built man of his time.

NEW RULE #11 • You'll get better results working your ass off on a bad program than you will loafing through a good program.

Every now and then, those workouts you see in the bodybuilding magazines are real. That is, the bodybuilders actually do them, and have muscles to show for them. And the more real they are, in many cases, the more they suck. That's when a careful reader realizes, to his horror, that bad programs can build huge muscles. Insiders will tell you that the biggest bodybuilders have rare genetics that allow them to grow from any combination of serious lifting and the right chemicals. What is seriously lifted, and how it's lifted, matters less for these rare beasts than outsiders would ever suspect.

Even the genetically average drug-free lifter will get good results from lousy programs with enough hard work and tolerance for pain. (The worse the program, the greater the pain.)

Training hard and consistently is the key to making gains on a good or bad system. The difference, as Alwyn says, is that a good program is "almost magical" when you put in the effort to make it work. In other words, if you put forth the same effort in a good program as you would in a bad program, you'll get much better results from the good program, and with a much lower injury risk.

But without the effort, the best program is only as valuable as the paper it's written on.

NEW RULE #12 • Fast lifting is not more dangerous than slow lifting.

This seems like an obscure point to make here, in this chapter, but I have a reason for talking about this up front. As you'll learn below, most periodized workout systems include at least a short phase devoted to fast lifting. That's because muscle power— the ability to move an object, or your body, at maximum velocity—is important. Power not only has real-life uses, as I explained in Chapter 1; it has what I consider underrated muscle-building properties.

But I'll get into that below. What I want to stress here is the safety issue. For as long as I've been a fitness journalist, and probably for at least a decade before that, every person who sets foot in a commercial gym has been told that lifting slowly is safe and lifting fast is dangerous.

Words like "ballistic" and "jerking" make fast lifting sound like bad sex. It's a wonder the Olympic lifts haven't been given more sinister names, like "oozing pustule" and "confiscatory taxation."

Meanwhile, words like "slow" and "smooth" are equated not just with good lifting, but good loving.

The only problem is that the conventional wisdom is wrong.

Fast lifting isn't inherently dangerous, if you're talking about a real exercise performed correctly by someone who's properly prepared to do that lift. (A lot of caveats, I know, but not enough to rule out fast lifting for healthy guys.) And slow lifting isn't always safe. In fact, in some circumstances, working at unnaturally slow speeds can be more dangerous than working at normal, faster speeds.

This is from Stuart McGill** in *Low Back Disorders*: "The instruction to always lift a load smoothly may not invariably result in the least risk of injury." The longer a muscle stays under tension, McGill writes, the greater the risk that it'll deform. In fact, your muscles and connective tissues have a property called viscoelasticity, which allows them to perform a fast movement without injury. But the same movement performed slowly might cause a strain or tear, since the muscles and connective tissues have more chance to deform.

That's why our instincts tell us to lift some objects quickly and some slowly. But if we go against our instincts and try to lift everything at the same slow, smooth pace, we may be putting our most vulnerable joints at unnecessary risk of injury.

I'm not saying that fast lifting is universally safe and always the best option. Beginners, for example, should start with lifts that can be done safely at a deliberate speed. Even intermediate and advanced lifters need to work up to fast lifts, if they've never done them before.

But that's why we use periodization to design good workout programs. And with no further rules for you to learn, I'll be happy to walk you through it.

THE BEST DESIGN FOR LIFTING, PERIOD

"Periodization" means something very simple: planned changes in training programs in order to get steady improvements. Key words: *planned* changes, *steady* improvements.

The idea of periodized workout programs started with athletic training, and it followed a pretty simple and logical model based on three stages: pre-season, in-season, off-season.

Let's say you're a college basketball player. Your season is November to March, more or less. Let's say your pre-season workouts start in June. From June through October, you'll steadily increase the *intensity* of your workouts, both in the weight room and on the basketball court. You'll also focus more of your effort on improving your *skill*, since that's most crucial to success.

But at the same time, you'll steadily decrease the *volume* of your workouts. In other words, you'll start off doing a lot of exercise, but at a low intensity and requiring little skill. Then, as you crank up the intensity and the focus on high-level, sport-specific skills, you'll steadily lower the volume. You're working harder, so your body can't do as much total work without breaking down.

When you start your season, you'll continue along the same paths—higher intensity, lower volume—until you get to the major tournaments. At that point, you drop the intensity of your training and the focus on skills in practice, because performance in competition is all that matters now. You don't want to leave anything in the weight room that you can use on the court.

The end of your season brings an end to serious training. The off-season is for recovery, mental as well as physical. You can and should still play basketball. You can and should still work in the weight room. But you do those things at your own speed, letting your body tell you what it can and can't do.

Two months later, you go into your pre-season workouts and start the next periodization cycle.

PERIODIZATION FOR GYM RATS

Here's a question you may have at this point: What the hell does this have to do with me? And it's a fair question. After all, if you've been training for a few years, you probably haven't periodized anything—you simply go to the gym three or four or five or six days a week, and lift the best way you know how. You change your workouts when you learn something new.

And if you've never lifted before, or tried but failed to stick with a program, you may wonder how you can commit to a year-long program when the first month usually presents challenge enough.

Without knowing it, you've presented the best possible arguments for periodizing your programs.

The consistent lifter probably hasn't made consistent gains—it's all been start-stop. Ask me if you can name this tune:

1. You start off great guns and make gains for a month or two.
2. You stop making gains but continue for a few more weeks on the same program, perhaps adding sets or exercises to get things moving forward again.
3. You don't make the gains, and your motivation wavers. You start to backslide a bit.
4. You discover a new workout technique, or some new exercises, and suddenly you're motivated again and making new gains.
5. Repeat as necessary.

Periodization (and yes, I find the word kind of annoying, too) gets you out of this cycle by figuring out in advance when you'll need to shake up your program. A well-designed workout program will start you off with higher-volume, lower-intensity, lower-skill workouts, then gradually push you toward heavier weights, lower repetitions, and exercises that require more skill.

In other words, the fun stuff.

Now, about that beginner or constant re-starter: My guess is that you'll find it easier to stick with a program that regularly changes, as opposed to one that offers the same stuff week after week, stuff that you find boring after the first few workouts. Speaking as a lifelong lifter, I know I get a little extra adrenaline surge when I know I'm going to try something different in that day's workout. You may think I'm nuts, but my guess is that you'll soon find yourself charged up by the new, too.

THE FIVE-STAGE ROCKET

You can find any number of ways to periodize programs, but here's the one that's considered "classic" periodization. (It's not exactly what Alwyn uses in the *New Rules* workouts; that's a modification called "undulating periodization," and I explain it below.)

Stage 1: Anatomical adaptation

More big words, but you could also say "general conditioning" or "getting your ass in some semblance of shape" and still be talking about the same thing.

This period gives you a fairly high volume of exercise, with the idea that you'll develop some strength and some muscle mass, but mostly you'll condition your muscles and connective tissues. Not only will they have more endurance, they'll be fully prepared for the heavier work to follow.

Stage 2: Hypertrophy

This word (hy-PURR-truh-fee) is easier to remember if you keep in mind that it's the opposite of "atrophy." You want your muscles to get bigger here. That means you'll be working with heavier weights than you did in Stage 1, and doing fewer repetitions, usually eight to twelve per set. You're still doing a lot of work, but this time with more focus on making bigger muscles, as opposed to better-conditioned muscles.

If you recall the section in Chapter 3 that talked about the ideal rep range for muscle growth, you know this is it. The mechanism at work here is often referred to as "time under tension," a theory that suggests the longer you can keep muscles under a high level of tension, the more they'll grow.

An important distinction: You aren't working with maximum weights here; if the workout chart tells you to do eight reps at a normal tempo, that means you're taking about three or four seconds per repetition—one second to lift, a very brief pause, and another second or two to lower the weight. If you were going for max weight, you'd lift faster than that. So your goal is to use a weight that allows you to complete the designated repetitions at the designated speed. (I'll explain the use of different lifting speeds in detail in Part 4.) The weight should feel damned heavy in the final reps, but the object here isn't to push yourself to any sort of limit; it's to *get ready* to push yourself. There's a big difference. This stage is about steady gains, not peak performance.

Stage 3: Strength

"Strength" is one of my favorite words in the English language. It means just about the same thing to everybody. And even in a field where everyone disagrees about everything, there's some consensus on how best to build it.

In this stage, we're still dropping reps, still increasing weights, while doing more sets. We're also lifting faster. We're no longer trying to build bigger muscles by keeping them under tension longer; we're moving toward maximum tension within the muscles.

Stage 4: Maximal strength/power

Two simple definitions: *Strength* is the ability to move a weight, regardless of how fast you move it. *Power* is the ability to move a weight fast.

Tension Deficit

If you see a phrase like "time under tension," you probably think it refers to grocery shopping with young kids. (Especially if you screw up and wander down the candy aisle, a mistake few of us parental commandos make more than once.) But in the past few years, "time under tension," as it applies to strength training, has been elevated to an exalted status, the key to all that heaven will allow.

Well, bigger muscles, anyway.

Here's the idea:

1. Muscles only grow when they're subjected to a certain threshold of tension—that is, they have to be under some kind of strain to grow.

2. Momentary tension, however high, doesn't produce bigger muscles with any certainty. And high momentary tension—from a maximum bench press, for example—is far more dangerous than continuous tension.

3. Continuous tension, thus, is the key to muscle growth.

4. There is an optimal amount of time that muscles need to be under tension to produce growth.

The way "time under tension" (TUT) is used in bodybuilding articles, you'd think that it has solid science behind it.

Nope.

Nobody knows if the theory is right or wrong, since, to my knowledge, no studies have compared different times under tension to see which produces bigger muscles.

The late *Supertraining* author, Mel Siff,** used to argue that you couldn't measure it accurately in any case, since muscles aren't really under continuous tension during a repetition. The amount of tension varies according to the speed of the lift, the speed of the lowering, and the length of the pauses in between lifting and lowering. And there's no friggin' way in hell you could control for all that in a scientific study. People aren't machines—they can't knock out rep after rep in which, say, the lift takes exactly two seconds, the pause at the top is exactly one second, the lowering takes exactly four seconds, and the pause at the bottom is exactly one second.

If you could find a way to get a human to do repetitions that are exactly eight seconds long, and compare eight reps of those to eight reps done at a normal speed, the results would still depend on the amount of weight lifted and the speed at which it's lifted. In other words, to what do you compare it? To a lifter using a lighter weight and banging out the eight reps as fast as possible? To a guy choosing the heaviest possible weight and grinding out eight reps at varying speeds (faster at first, slower at the end)?

None of this proves the TUT touters wrong, and that's why Alwyn's *New Rules* workouts include a range of lifting speeds, which is just one of many variables he uses to induce gains in strength and muscle size. At the end, you won't be able to tell if your gains had anything to do with TUT. But then again, who cares? You're still bigger and stronger.

So let's take two guys who can each bench-press 200 pounds. Let's make them identical twins, with the exact same arm length. So if you put the two of them up against each other in a display of strength and power, their strength would be exactly the same. But let's say one twin can lift the 200 pounds faster than the other. That twin has more power, since he can lift the same weight the same distance, but do it faster.

Power, unlike strength, isn't easily measurable. And to make it all the more confusing, the athletes who achieve the most success in sports involving maximum power (football, say) are also the strongest. Back in 1991, William Kraemer** and Andy Fry** looked at college football players in Division I, Division II, and Division III. If you assume that Division I players (the guys who would play at brand-name schools like Notre Dame, Michigan, and Oklahoma) are better than the guys in Division II, who are better than the guys in Division III, then it's significant that the higher-division guys are stronger than the lower-division guys.

Their strength, in other words, has to be considered a major reason why they're better than the guys in whatever division is below them. And, turning it around, a guy who's in Division III is there, in large part, because he's not as strong as the average player in Division II.

Other research has shown that starters in Division I schools are stronger than reserves.

The same held true with studies of throwers in track and field events. The best shot-putters and discus throwers could also squat and bench-press more than the guys they beat in throwing competitions.

But: It's really impossible to distinguish "strength" and "power" in these studies, since an exercise called the power clean is part of the equation. The "power clean" is more like an Olympic lift than something you'd see in a powerlifting competition. (And, just to make it more brain-splittingly confusing, the term "powerlifting" is really inaccurate. The three lifts—squat, bench press, deadlift—are tests of strength, not power.) You start with a bar on the ground, then pull it to your shoulders. The lift combines slow and fast elements, but the fast part is the hard part. So it's more a test of power than strength.

I think the most reasonable conclusion is that strength and power are closely related and, in combination, absolutely correlate to the ability to generate force on the athletic field.

That's why you have a combined strength-power phase, as opposed to a pure-power phase, featuring nothing but fast, Olympic-type lifts with weights that would be easy for you to lift slowly.

Stage 5: Recovery

This can be a week or two without training. Or it can be a couple months of mostly unstructured workouts. That is, you go into the gym, you do your favorite exercises, and you don't put pressure on yourself to reach certain goals. Or it can be a structured program in which you work on rehabilitating an injury under professional supervision.

MY PERIODIZATION HAS A FIRST NAME . . .

It should come as no surprise that, if periodization in general is a good idea for athletes and gym rats alike, someone would come up with more sophisticated forms of it. Once again, I'm going to hit you with some multisyllabic terms that aren't particularly sexy. (You wouldn't whisper "conjugate periodization" to someone you hoped to get conjugal with, to state the obvious.)

But if you understand the ideas, you understand why Alwyn designed the *New Rules* programs the way he did. If you don't, you'll get lost.

And once you're lost, it's just one short step back to the world of endless biceps curls and leg extensions.

One more reassurance: The ideas behind Alwyn's workouts are complex and sophisticated, and they represent the very latest in scientific understanding of how muscles get bigger and stronger. But the workouts themselves aren't difficult to understand or execute. So, while I want you to understand the "why," you'll be surprised at how simple the "what" can be.

Linear periodization

This is what I described above: You do this, progress to that, progress to the next thing, get to a peak, and back off. Linear periodization means never having to say you're doing the same workout you did last month. And, while it's better than the average divide-and-conquer bodybuilding program, it's not always the best plan.

"The main problem with linear periodization is that you constantly move away from the quality you've just developed," Alwyn says. For example, in one stage you develop muscular endurance, then steadily progress toward heavier lifts, with fewer reps, thus losing some of the endurance you worked to improve. "So if it was important to develop that quality in the first place, why not at least maintain it?"

That's why some more sophisticated periodization systems have emerged. The key to them is that they improve on what periodization does best—help you build strength, power, and muscle mass—without taking an all-or-nothing approach to each phase of your program.

Alwyn uses these three types of periodization in the *New Rules* programs:

Alternating periodization

You'll find this in the Fat-Loss program. You can probably guess what it is by the name: In Stage 1, Alwyn has you doing sets of ten to twelve repetitions, mostly. In Stage 2, you go a little heavier, with sets of eight to ten. Then, in Stage 3, you go up as high as twenty reps per set, with an average of thirteen to fourteen per set.

In other words, instead of going in a straight line from the highest reps to the lowest, you shake up your metabolism by alternating from medium to low to high in the three stages.

Conjugate periodization

With linear periodization, you lift pretty light weights for high repetitions in the early stages, then heavy weights for low reps in the later stages. But where is it written that you can't mix and match?

That's the idea behind conjugate periodization—each program combines some heavy lifts for strength, some fast lifts for power, some medium-rep sets for muscle growth, and some high-rep sets for muscular endurance and overall conditioning.

For example, in the Strength II program, Alwyn has you do two heavy sets of four squats for pure strength, followed by an eight-rep set for muscle growth, followed by a twelve-rep set for muscle endurance. (I'll explain all this in more detail in Chapter 20.)

Undulating periodization

Classic, linear periodization assumes that every athlete in training has a specific moment in his season when he needs to reach a peak. But few sports really work that way. Take basketball: If the players only peak at tournament time, then that means they're playing at less than their peak throughout the season, which could keep them from reaching the post-season tournaments in the first place.

So strength coaches created a different model, called "undulating periodization," in which the athletes are able to maintain high levels of muscle endurance, strength, and mass throughout the season. But it's more than a maintenance program. In fact, some new research shows that undulating programs develop strength and size faster than linear systems.

Consider this study in the May 2002 issue of the *Journal of Strength and Conditioning Research*: The researchers took a group of college-age lifters with an average of five years' training experience. Half did a linear program—three sets of eight reps one month, three sets of six the next, three sets of four the last. The other group did something called "daily undulating periodization" (or DUP, surely among the most unfortunate acronyms in the entire language). They did three sets of eight on Monday, three sets of six on Wednesday, and three sets of four on Friday. So they did the same program for three months, but they never did the same protocol twice in a week.

The linear group still had big gains—average increases of 14.4 percent in the bench press and 25.7 percent in the leg press. But the DUP group doubled them up—28.8 percent in the bench and 55.8 percent in the leg press.

That's not exactly the way Alwyn uses undulating periodization in the *New Rules* hypertrophy workouts, but it shows the power of shaking things up.

All these variations on linear periodization are still fairly new, and research hasn't yet established that they're always better than linear systems, or which variations might be better than others. However, plenty of research has shown that periodization, of any type, isn't just better than other types of programs. It's *dramatically* better.

5

Warming Up

You could divide all lifters into two groups, based on how they warm up:

Group 1 gets on a treadmill or stationary bike and stays there for somewhere between fifteen and thirty minutes. I'm not sure how anyone in this group arrives at the optimum time to tread or cycle, but I suspect it has something to do with the length of the magazine articles they're reading or the segment on CNN on the TV overhead.

Group 2 loads up a barbell and starts lifting.

Now, the people in Group 1 may literally get warm, but they don't do anything to prepare their bodies to lift weights. And when they do finally get around to lifting, they tend to do it about as intensely as they pedaled that bike. (Remember New Rule #7: Don't "do the machines.")

The people in Group 2 tend to be the most serious, hardest-working lifters in the gym. (And I should note that they're often a lot stronger than I am.) But they don't do anything special to prepare their bodies for lifting, either. I've seen these guys walk in and start lifting with 90 percent of the maximum weight they're going to use on that exercise.

I hope to get two ideas across in this chapter:

1. You will lift better, with less risk of injury, if you take a few minutes to prepare your body for the task.
2. Walking on a treadmill or riding a stationary bike doesn't prepare your body for the task of lifting heavy weights.

First, though, I must rule:

NEW RULE #13 ● A good warm-up doesn't have to make your body warm.

At least, not all of it. The idea is to make the right parts warm. Studies in the 1980s and '90s showed that warm muscles are less likely to tear. That is, a slightly warmer muscle is less stiff, and a less-stiff muscle has less resistance to force. So when you do a heavy lift with warm rather than unprepared lower-body muscles, you're less likely to hurt the targeted muscles and connective tissues.

The problem with saying what I just said, though, is that it's stunningly obvious, and you didn't buy a book with "New Rules" in the title so you could learn what the guy cleaning mirrors at your neighborhood McGym could've told you.

Here's what he doesn't know (which I'm pulling from *Supertraining*, by the late Mel Siff**).

- Research in the 1950s showed that low-intensity warm-ups don't improve strength performance. In other words, jogging on the treadmill may warm up your lower-body muscles, but it doesn't prepare them for heavy squats.
- The more intense the exercise you're about to do, the more you need a warm-up. The converse is also true: If you're doing easy, low-intensity stuff, you don't need to warm up for it. (Although it's fine if you do.)
- The better a lifter you are, the more you get out of a warm-up.
- The more similar the warm-up activities are to the lifts for which you're preparing, the better they'll work.

NEW RULE #14 ● Stretching is not a warm-up.

I'm going to get into this more in the next chapter, but for now, I just want to separate the discussions. There's no evidence that pre-exercise stretching prevents injuries or improves strength or power. In fact, there's a growing body of evidence suggesting that pre-exercise stretching *inhibits* power performance.

So when I talk about warming up here, I'm not talking about stretching. Some of the exercises in this chapter do stretch your muscles, but there's nothing about increasing the length of muscle tissues *before a workout* that makes you stronger or better prepared to lift.

WARM, IF NOT FUZZY

I have dozens of fitness books on my shelves, and I frequently consult six or seven of them for my articles and books. These books tell you everything you'd ever want to know about how muscles are built, how exercises should be performed, and how those muscles and exercises can be used to become a better athlete.

Most of them, though, don't say squat about warm-ups. I mean *nothing*. Not even a mention in the index.

And when they do talk about warming up, it tends to be stuff you probably already know. Take, for example, *Essentials of Strength Training and Conditioning*. It's the official textbook of the National Strength and Conditioning Association. You have to practically memorize the thing to become certified as a trainer by the NSCA, as Alwyn and I are. In a twenty-two-page chapter titled "Stretching and Warm-up," *Essentials* expends less than half a page on warming up.

Scandalous?

No, just indicative of how boring a subject this is, even for academics who write textbooks, a specific breed of infogeek that ordinarily displays a nearly bottomless well of tedium tolerance. I mean, there's a reason why the majority of studies I mention in this chapter took place before most of us were born. All the important questions had already been answered.

So I'll make this quick.

Let's assume there are three types of warm-up exercise:

GENERAL WARM-UPS are things like walking, jogging, and bike-riding. They're low-intensity, and they help you get the creaks out of your joints. (Joints are naturally lubricated by a bodily secretion called synovial fluid. As you warm up, the fluid spreads over the joint, acting as a lubricant to decrease friction.) But if you overdo them, you end up burning off energy supplies that could be better used during the actual workout. Rule of thumb? Five to ten minutes, tops, for a general warm-up. More than that, and you're probably wasting time and energy.

SEMI-SPECIFIC WARM-UPS (a term I believe I just made up) include exercises like the ones Alwyn recommends later in this chapter. In *Core Performance*, Mark Verstegen calls this category of exercise "movement prep." The idea is to put your muscles through a series of drills that challenge them to stretch and contract. Even though these preparatory movements don't precisely mimic weight-lifting exercises, they do wake up the muscles and nerves so they'll be better at those exercises when you get to them.

SPECIFIC WARM-UPS involve practicing the exercises you're going to do right before you do them. So the squat is a specific warm-up for . . . the squat.

The amount of weight you use in a specific warm-up, and the number of repetitions, is really a matter of your own comfort and training style. If there's a rule that applies in every case, I haven't seen it. But here's a general guideline Alwyn uses with his clients (and which I've used for years without knowing anyone else did it that way):

Do one warm-up set for every fifty pounds of weight you want to lift in your first work set. (In the *New Rules* workouts, starting on page 202, we don't list warm-up sets. So every set on the chart is a "work" set.)

As for repetitions, you want to start with roughly half the number you'll do in that first work set, and then reduce a repetition in every subsequent warm-up set.

Let's say you're going to do a set of ten squats with 150 pounds. Here's how you'd warm up:

1. Warm-up set #1: 50 pounds, 5 reps
2. Warm-up set #2: 100 pounds, 4 reps

You don't have to hit these precise numbers. An Olympic barbell weighs forty-five pounds, so you could simply use the unloaded bar for five reps for the first warm-up set. For the second, you could use ninety-five, since that's easy to set up—it's just the forty-five-pound bar, plus a twenty-five-pound weight plate on each side.

You may wonder why you don't do a set of ten reps to warm up for a set of ten reps. The answer: You want your muscles to practice the movement, but you don't want to exhaust them. And high repetitions, even with light weights, do expend some of the fuel in your muscles, which can be better used in the work sets. (Fun fact: It takes about eight minutes to restore 97 percent of the phosphocreatine in your muscles; this is the material that produces energy for short, intense efforts, including most weight-lifting sets. I'm not saying that lifting light weights will burn off significant amounts of phosphocreatine, but it does illustrate how carefully you have to guard it.)

Now let's say you're an advanced lifter, and you're warming up for multiple sets of three reps with 300 pounds. Your strategy is similar. In this case, I'm going to use the "real" weights that someone would actually load on the bar, using twenty-five- and forty-five-pound plates, separately and in combination:

1. Warm-up set #1: 45 pounds, 5 reps
2. Warm-up set #2: 95 pounds, 4 reps
3. Warm-up set #3: 135 pounds, 3 reps (that's the bar, plus a 45-pound plate on each side)
4. Warm-up set #4: 185 pounds, 2 reps
5. Warm-up set #5: 225 pounds, 1 rep (that's the bar with two 45s on each side)
6. Warm-up set #6: 275 pounds, 1 rep

You don't have to rest any specified amount of time between warm-up sets. Alwyn says that the time it takes to change the weights and drink from your water bottle is plenty.

After the final warm-up set, take about two to three minutes, then tear into your work sets. And believe me, when you get to the point where you need to do six warm-up sets, you won't be in any mood to screw around. You'll make those inert hunks of iron pay for your annoyance.

Another question: Do you have to warm up like this for every exercise? I'll confess I don't. I'll warm up thoroughly and meticulously for lower-body exercises, like squats and deadlifts. By my standards, that means about five minutes of general warm-up, about five minutes of semi-specific exercises, and whatever it takes for my specific warm-up. Once I'm finished with my heavy lifts, I'll go straight to medium- or high-rep work sets without any more warm-up. I figure my joints are lubricated, my muscles are warm and primed for work, and any sets I do at that point should be results-oriented. (I can't remember the last time I hurt myself lifting, so I have to think it's working.)

For upper-body lifts, like bench presses, I follow the same protocol for specific warm-ups, but I don't do much in the way of general or semi-specific drills. During the winter, when I'm walking into the gym from the cold, I'll do a few minutes of general warm-up. But in the other three seasons, I usually go straight to the semi-specific and specific warm-ups.

THE SEMI-CHALLENGING, SEMI-SPECIFIC WARM-UP ROUTINE

Here's a five-move, semi-specific warm-up you can use before any workout:

✳ Walking lunge with upper-body twist

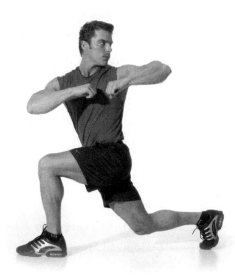

Prepares your body for lunging and twisting exercises; forces hip flexors, gluteals, and thigh muscles to stretch and contract while utilizing a horizontal twist.

➤ Take a long step forward with your left leg, and as you descend into the lunge position, twist your torso to the left. Then, without returning to the starting position, rise and take another long step forward with your right leg, and twist to your right. Do five to ten lunges with each leg.

✳ Lateral lunge with opposite-hand reach and touch

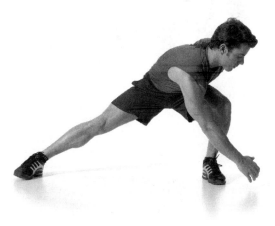

Further prepares body for lunging and twisting exercises, this time forcing inner-thigh and outer-thigh muscles to stretch and contract; utilizes a diagonal twist.

➤ Take a long step straight to the left, bending your left leg while keeping your right leg straight. Reach with your right hand and touch the floor on the outside of your left foot. (If you can't reach that far without discomfort, just do what you can.) Rise back to the starting position, then lunge to your right side, reaching with your left hand. Again, do five to ten to each side.

✳ **Ball bridge/Russian twist**

Bridge fires rear-body muscles—lower back, gluteals, hamstrings, calves, shoulder-blade muscles—while stretching chest, abdominals, and quadriceps. Russian twist works torso-rotating muscles, which were prepared in previous moves.

➤ Lie on your back on a Swiss ball so your shoulders are on the ball, your heels are on the floor, and your body forms a straight line from shoulders to heels. You want your arms straight out to your sides and perpendicular to your body. You should feel a good contraction in your gluteals and hamstrings. Hold for fifteen to thirty seconds.

➤ Then go to a Russian twist: Your shoulders are on the ball, with your arms reaching straight out in front of your chest and your hands together. Your knees are bent and your feet are flat on the floor. Raise your hips, so your body forms a straight line from shoulders to knees. Now twist your upper body to the left, with your head turning so your eyes follow your hands. Return to the starting position, and repeat to your right side. Keep your lower body as motionless as possible. Do five to ten reps to each side.

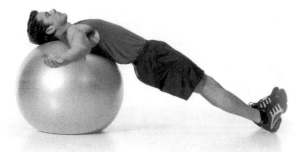

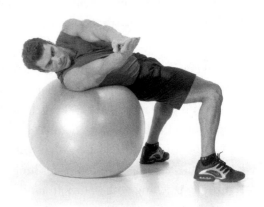

✳ Inchworm

"Wakes up" torso-stabilizing muscles in midsection and upper back while stretching gluteals, hamstrings, and calves.

➤ Stand with your feet together, hands on the floor. Slowly walk your hands forward until your body is as elongated as you can make it, with your weight balanced on your toes and hands. Now walk your feet back up to your hands until your feet and hands are both flat on the floor again. Do five or six of these.

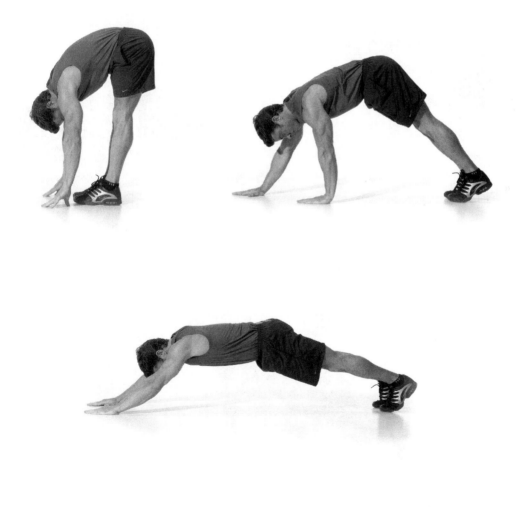

✴ T-push-up

Activates front-torso muscles in chest and shoulders while working torso-stabilizing muscles from upper to lower back.

➤ Get into push-up position—your hands directly beneath your shoulders, your body straight from neck to ankles. Lower your chest to the floor, then pivot to your left side as you push back up, with your left arm straight up over your left shoulder and perpendicular to the floor. Your body should form the letter T (lowercase). Pivot back, lower your chest to the floor again, then pivot to the right as you push yourself back up. Do five or six T-push-ups to each side.

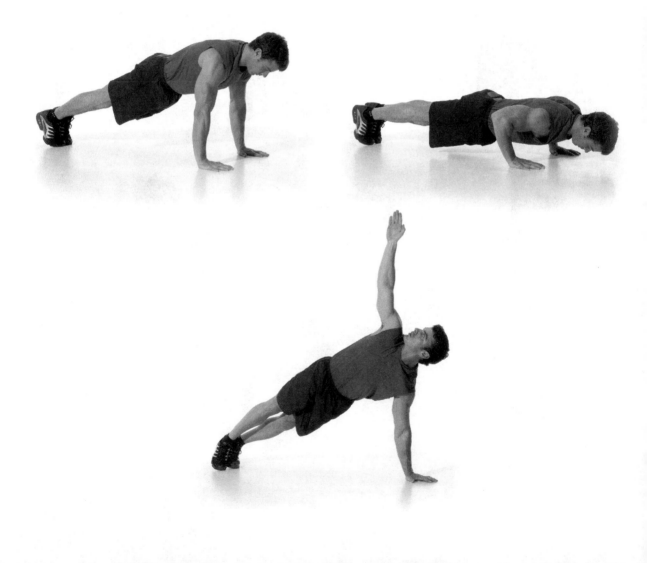

Flexibility

6

EXPERTS FALL ALL OVER themselves arguing over the importance of flexibility, the possible downsides of stretching exercises (particularly before an athletic event in which someone needs to generate maximum power), the best ways to stretch. There's only one constant: Every strength and conditioning coach in the world uses flexibility exercises with his athletes.

I'll tell you why, right after I rule.

NEW RULE #15 • You don't need to warm up to stretch.

In Chapter 5, I said that stretching isn't a good warm-up. Now I want to point out that you don't have to go through a good warm-up if you want to stretch. Unless you wake up in the morning and try to put your foot behind your head—and why would you?—you don't have to worry about hurting yourself.

Studies have shown that you get a greater range of motion when you stretch after warming up. But that doesn't mean you hurt yourself stretching if you don't warm up first.

If you feel like stretching, stretch.

NEW RULE #16 ● Lifting by itself may increase your flexibility.

As a general rule, active people are more flexible than inactive ones. Put another way, anyone who gets up and moves will have better range of motion in his joints than someone who doesn't. Sitting—whether at work, in a car, or in your cell on death row—will tend to lead to a shortening of two muscle groups: the hip flexors (the strips of muscle on the front of the pelvis) and the chest and shoulder muscles involved in pushing exercises. Your hip flexors are always shortened when you sit, and the front-torso muscles surrounding your shoulder joints tend to shorten when you slump forward, or reach out to hold the steering wheel, or type on your laptop.

Conversely, the muscles on the back of your body tend to get overstretched.

Almost any form of exercise requires good posture, which means you pull your shoulders back. And almost any sports- or fitness-related movement involves long strides that will help your hip flexors reach their optimal length.

Thus, most people who exercise are at least a bit more flexible than those who don't.

Weight lifting used to get a bad rap when it came to flexibility. The idea was that all those icky muscles made someone "muscle-bound" and thus less flexible than the admirably nonmuscular population. Of course, that's total horsecrap.

Rude Awakening

Some of us like to work out in the morning, some at midday, some in the evening. But all of us should avoid doing anything that involves bending and twisting in the first hour after awakening. That's because our spinal discs fill with fluid overnight, according to Stuart McGill** in *Ultimate Back Fitness and Performance*.

McGill says the extra fluid magnifies whatever stresses we put on those discs. Heavy stretching, as well as heavy lifting, is a pretty bad idea.

The discs lose 90 percent of that accumulated fluid within the first hour after rising, McGill writes, which means you should be perfectly safe if you wait sixty minutes to lift or stretch.

The first study debunking the notion of muscle binding came out in 1956, and numerous studies since then have further refined the idea. Typically, strength training increases ankle flexibility and shoulder mobility in some, but not all, directions. The type of strength training matters, too: Olympic weight lifters are extremely flexible—right up there with gymnasts—while powerlifters tend to have limited shoulder-joint mobility. Part of that is due to the size of their chest muscles, and part is task-specific. That is, they need stiffer shoulder joints to bench-press as much weight as possible.

The best strategy for gaining muscle while increasing your flexibility is lifting through a full range of motion. Don't stop a squat or shoulder press short in either direction, even though you can lift more weight when you don't have to move it as far. Limited ranges have their place, especially during heavy-duty, strength-focused periods. But in the long run, you want to move your muscles through the entire range.

Another important factor is balanced training—equal volume and intensity for muscles on the front and rear of your body. Most of us naturally have strength imbalances from front to back and left to right. These even out over time with a good training system, such as Alwyn's *New Rules* workouts. The last thing you want is to exacerbate the problem with unbalanced workouts focused on the "mirror muscles" on the front of your body.

LET'S NOT STRETCH THE TRUTH

Research on stretching is highly equivocal. That is, you can find a study to support just about any position you want to take. And the research often uses extreme stretching protocols—holding one stretch for ten minutes, for example—that have no relationship to what you or I might do in the gym.

Still, I think there are some conclusions you can draw, if you combine what we learn from research with what forward-thinking trainers and strength coaches like Alwyn learn by experience.

Most important, Alwyn has told me, is to make a distinction between "stretching" and "flexibility training." He may have clients stretch to develop flexibility, but he'd never assume that everyone needs to stretch for the sake of stretching.

The difference between the two is more than mere semantics. Most people think of stretching as something that changes the structure of muscles and connective tissues, making them longer. But tendons (the connective tissues that attach muscles to bones) have very little ability to lengthen.

They can get stronger and stiffer through strength training and then more pliable through a variety of exercises that take them through a full range of motion. But they won't get much longer through stretching exercises. Nor will the bellies of the muscles change length or shape. The only way to make them longer is to induce some kind of injury (medieval dungeon-masters were said to be very good at this), and that negates the point of exercise.

It helps to look at flexibility as something that happens in the nerves as much as in the muscles and joints. When certain structures within your muscles—things with exotic names like "Pacinian corpuscles," "muscle spindles," and "Golgi tendon organs"—realize that some part of your body is trying to stretch, they quickly assess the challenge and render a verdict: "Yes, we're going to allow this," or "No, this moron is trying to get us all killed and he must be stopped."

If it's the latter, then those structures signal your muscles to tighten up, in effect forbidding a stretch beyond your safety zones. (These same mechanisms can inhibit strength, if they sense you're trying to lift something too heavy. More on that in Chapter 20.)

Your individual safety zones are determined by a long list of factors:

- *your fitness level* (the better shape you're in, the more range of motion your nervous system will allow)
- *injury status* (these mechanisms will always try to prevent further injury, even if it means shortening your range of motion and thus producing the potential for more injuries down the road)
- *muscle imbalances* (if you overdevelop one set of muscles, they'll be tighter than the muscles that perform the opposing actions)
- *gender* (women are more flexible by nature, but you already knew that)
- *genetics* (you're more flexible than some, less flexible than others, and no amount of stretching will change the individual structure of your joints or the length of your connective tissues)

Another factor is the size of your muscles. One time, at a magazine photo shoot I supervised, the two very fit models couldn't do some yoga-type move that involved intertwining arms in front of the chest. They were just too damned big for the exercise. I could get a little closer to the final position than they could, but only because I have smaller arm and chest muscles. The women at the shoot, on the other hand, had no trouble with it.

FLEX TIME

The key to increased flexibility is coaxing those structures, those corpuscles and spindles and tendon organs, into allowing a greater range of motion. It's like when you were a teenager and trying to get your parents to let you borrow their car on Saturday night: First you had to prove you could make it out of the driveway without running over the mailbox.

That will come with general conditioning, including basic exercises through a full range of motion.

Another flex factor is coordination—muscle control. As you get better at exercises, particularly as you get better at controlling the stabilizing muscles on any given lift, your nervous system will allow greater flexibility.

As you may have guessed, I'm pretty lukewarm on the subject of traditional flexibility exercises, what we call "static" stretches. I don't like or dislike them. They're useful sometimes, but if you're flexible enough to do all the exercises in this program, I don't see why you'd need to do all that extra work. As Alwyn said, there's no point in increasing flexibility for its own sake.

How much flexibility is enough? I think you should be flexible enough to do the six basic movements in this program—squat, deadlift, lunge, push, pull, twist—with perfect form. Any level of flexibility that falls short of this standard is unacceptable, but any level beyond that is a bonus.

The Aerobics Myth

I HAVE A BIAS against endurance exercise. In my defense, I developed it the hard way, having tried multiple times, dating back to my freshman year of high school, to develop better endurance. Each time I failed to reach that goal, and failed to enjoy the process.

My last attempt was in 1999. I was working in an office in which everyone was a runner, and I was the only guy who focused exclusively on strength training.

So I launched a running program with a big-bodied coworker, the only guy in the office who wouldn't leave me in the dust after a quarter-mile. As usual, it was a disaster for me; I lost strength and muscle, my knees ached continually, and I found I couldn't develop my endurance beyond a certain point, which was only slightly beyond my starting level. On top of that, I felt like crap. My body was generating the opposite of pleasure-causing endorphins. (I dubbed them "endurephins"—they made every minute of exercise miserable to endure.)

There's a happy ending: I felt better as soon as I quit running and have never been tempted to resume.

My experience with endurance exercise doesn't mean it won't work for you. Even when I'm at my most overbearing as an advocate of strength training, I don't want anyone to quit running or swimming if they enjoy those things. Remember my first two rules of exercise: "Do something," and "Do something you like."

The more I write about fitness, the more I think that all types of exercise get you to more or less the same place: You feel better, and you improve your health. No, you can't train your body to lift heavy weights and expect to be able to run a marathon. No, you can't run an hour a day and expect to look like a bodybuilder. No, you can't limit your routine to three yoga classes a week and expect to look or perform like anything except a guy who takes three yoga classes a week.

The physiological adaptations to each type of exercise are going to be different, but the value of each may end up equal. Movement is good. Stress reduction is good. Weight control is good. Just getting away from your e-mail and cell phone for an hour a day is good. You can accomplish all that with weight lifting, running, pick-up basketball, Pilates, tennis, swimming, cycling, calisthenics, yoga, or just about anything else that qualifies as serious exercise.

But I'm not writing a book about running or pick-up basketball. And I'd rather cut off my chakras than write about yoga.

This book is about lifting—lifting for strength, lifting for muscle mass, lifting for fat loss, lifting for health, lifting for aesthetic appeal.

And yet, I'd be doing you a disservice if I didn't at least discuss endurance exercise. I've met plenty of lifters who don't like it, and I've certainly come across many who don't participate in it unless their car breaks down and there's no other way to get to the gym. But I don't think I've ever met a lifter who didn't think he was *supposed* to do it.

So let me rule a bit, and then I'll share with you our take (well, mostly Alwyn's take) on the role of endurance exercise in a lifter's training program.

NEW RULE #17 • Aerobic fitness is not a matter of life and death.

If you spend a lot of time reading scientific research, you'll notice that the phrase "exercise training" always means "endurance training." That's because there's still a pervasive idea in the world of exercise science, as well as among the general public, that movement designed to take you long distances is "real" exercise, and strength training is something different.

Embedded in the phrase is the idea that only endurance exercise improves health and contributes to a longer life.

So consider the results from a study of nearly 2,000 middle-aged men in the United Kingdom. The researchers, starting in 1979, looked at the subjects' exercise patterns and work-related physical activity (whether they lifted boxes on a loading dock or sat in an office all day, for example). They tracked the men until 1997.

The results, published in the journal *Heart* in 2003, found something that'll probably surprise you:

Light and moderate physical activity—walking, gardening, dancing, playing golf, bowling—had no effect on heart disease, death from heart disease, or death from all causes. Even the ones who did the most light and moderate activity, up to ninety minutes a day of walking or light yard work, got no measurable protection from heart disease or any other terminal illness.

The ones who got that protection were the ones who did what the researchers call "heavy" exercise: climbing stairs, playing vigorous start-stop sports like tennis and badminton, hiking, jogging, swimming, serious landscaping work. (Weight lifting wasn't included, for reasons I'll explain in a moment.)

But that's not only the surprising finding of the study:

The ones who got this protection—and we're only talking about one-fifth of the men studied—burned *as little as fifty-four calories a day* doing that heavy exercise. To put that in perspective, if you're a 180-pound guy, you'll burn just under 500 calories in an hour of chopping wood or shoveling snow (or serious weight lifting, for that matter). That's about seventy calories a day.

So one hour of heavy exercise a week offers you more protection from heart disease, as well as from death by any cause, than ninety minutes a day of walking.

Over the course of the study, the heavy-duty exercisers had 62 percent less chance of dying of heart disease and were 47 percent less likely to die of any cause than the rest of the men who participated.

Even those in the next group down, guys who were averaging between sixteen and fifty-three calories burned a day with heavy exercise, saw their chance of dying from any cause decline by 16 percent, while their risk of heart-related death dropped 27 percent.

My point here isn't that this study invalidates the idea of aerobic fitness as a path to health and longevity. I corresponded with one of the study authors, John W. G. Yarnell.** He emphasized that the men he and his colleagues studied lived in Caerphilly, a small town in southern Wales, and that the data were compiled in the 1980s, a time when few older men (forty-nine to sixty-four years old) would've been lifting weights. So almost all the "heavy" exercise included in the study had some endurance component.

Still, it doesn't take a lot of aerobic fitness to meet the fifty-four-calories-a-day standard. In fact, you wouldn't have to engage in any aerobic activities at all, since Dr. Yarnell's data include tennis and heavy yard work, which, as I'll explain below, don't primarily use the aerobic energy system for the "heavy" parts. An hour of serious yard work or home repair would do it. An hour of basketball or tennis or hockey or soccer would fill the bill.

Heck, by the standards we use today to determine exercise intensity, an hour of strength training would do it, even though I want to repeat that the men in Dr. Yarnell's study were not lifters.

Quick explanation:

Generally, "heavy" exercise means anything equal to or above six METs, or "metabolic equivalents." That means your metabolism cranks up to six times its resting speed to do the activity. Serious weight lifting is a six-MET activity, as are swimming (six to ten METs, depending on your effort), hiking (six), running (eight, at twelve-minute miles), cycling (six to ten), rowing (seven to twelve), cross-country skiing (seven to fourteen), tennis (five for doubles, up to eight for singles), basketball (six to eight), soccer (seven to ten), and dozens of others.

And, as suggested by the Caerphilly study, you can take your pick and help ward off death and heart disease.

NEW RULE #18 • You don't need to do endurance exercise to burn fat.

Visually, the idea that endurance exercise makes you lean seems irrefutable. Running burns calories. Runners tend to be thin. Case closed.

The converse of that idea also seems demonstrably true: Weight lifting doesn't burn as many calories as running, and weight lifters are often fat. Therefore, weight lifting can't possibly make you lean.

But then it all got muddled when people like me started writing about the metabolic effects of serious strength training. A tough weight workout cranks up your metabolism and can keep it elevated for up to two days afterward. The more muscle you build, the greater the effect.

On top of that, the muscle mass built from weight lifting boosts metabolism, over and above the effect of the workouts themselves. It's a relatively minor effect, and if you stop working out, you'll see how quickly your metabolism returns to whatever it was before. But it's an established fact that muscle mass is metabolically expensive—it takes extra calories to maintain.

We've also known for some time that endurance exercise doesn't increase metabolism beyond the calories burned during exercise, and those burned for a few hours afterward. (We exercise geeks call this "excess post-exercise oxygen consumption," or EPOC.)

So here's the bottom line on exercise and metabolism:

- Strength training cranks up metabolism for up to two days after a hard workout; the effect is magnified by any additional muscle mass you build.
- Endurance exercise doesn't increase post-workout metabolism aside from a short period after you finish.

All this is completely beside the point if your individual genetics don't allow you to gain a lot of muscle from strength training or if you don't want to work hard enough to elevate your metabolism. (You do have to push yourself to get that benefit. The studies showing dramatic metabolic boosts used workouts that are tougher than anything I do on a regular basis.)

And if you're good at endurance exercise, and do a lot of it every day, you don't need a huge metabolic boost to come out ahead. Let's say you have a 150-pound guy who runs an average of an hour a day, six days a week. His average speed is six miles an hour, or ten-minute miles. That's 680 calories a day, 4,080 a week. If you start off with a naturally fast metabolism, burning fat won't be an issue. You may worry more about the opposite situation—if you don't eat enough, you'll waste away.

My point in this New Rule, as it was in the previous rule, isn't to say that endurance exercise doesn't burn calories and help you control your weight. I just want to make the case that strength training can have the same effect, even if the mechanism is different.

Still better is the effect you get when you combine the right foods at the right times with the right workouts. That creates a higher "energy flux," a concept I'll explain in great detail in Part 5. Once you learn to manipulate energy flux, you'll have much more control over your body weight and much greater ability to reduce your body fat.

The Truth About Muscle and Metabolism

There's a lot of confusion about exercise, fat loss, and metabolism, and it's partly my fault. I've written that every pound of muscle you build increases your metabolism by up to fifty calories a day. Many others have written the same thing.

It's a great concept, and it would be even better if it were true.

I've only seen one study showing that "fifty calories per pound of muscle" result. It was a twenty-six-week study conducted at the University of Alabama–Birmingham, which found that older men and women (sixty-one to seventy-seven years old) got terrific results from a strength-training program. They added, on average, four and a half pounds of "lean mass" (mostly muscle, but also bone, blood, and anything else that isn't fat), without gaining any overall body weight.

Their body-fat percentages declined, their strength improved, and they burned a higher percentage of fat calories throughout the day (a calculation called "respiratory exchange ratio"). Fantastic results, right?

But here's where the "fifty calories per pound of muscle per day" figure came from: The subjects in the study, after twenty-six weeks, burned about eighty-seven more calories per day at rest (what we call "resting energy expenditure"). The researchers estimated that the subjects spent an extra thirty-seven minutes per day moving by the end of the study. Then they burned calories lifting weights three times a week. Finally, they expended a few extra calories digesting meals (this is called the "thermic effect of food," and I'll explain this is in detail in Part 5).

Add it up, and you get an average of 230 extra calories burned per day, or about 52 per pound of muscle they gained.

But less than half of those came from a measured increase in resting metabolism. The rest were exercise- or nutrition-related.

One time, I went through a pile of studies in my files, found three that measured metabolic rates in weight lifters, averaged the increases seen, and came up with a figure of about thirty-two calories per pound of muscle mass. That includes EPOC, or the extra calories your body burns a day or two after a tough workout.

Bottom line: It's the work you do, not the results of the work, that burns the extra calories.

NEW RULE #19 • When you combine serious strength training with serious endurance exercise, your body will probably choose endurance over muscle and strength.

Let's say you have a lot of time and energy on your hands and decide to lift weights for an hour at a time three days a week—Monday, Wednesday, Friday—and run an hour on Tuesday, Thursday, and Saturday. You'd think you would get the best of all worlds: bigger muscles, more strength, less fat, improved endurance.

But you'd be wrong. Chances are, your body would increase its strength and endurance. But muscle size would be compromised by what researchers call the "interference effect." That is, doing two opposing types of exercise (called "concurrent training") will interfere with each other, and your body will choose one or the other. In this case, your body will choose endurance over muscle growth, and strength and power may suffer as well.

The Greatest Program Ever

Every workout book ever published has promised more muscle and less fat. The more honest ones acknowledge that these two goals are nearly impossible to achieve at the same time, unless the person doing the workouts is an absolute beginner. The rest of us have to focus on one goal or the other at any given time.

Exercise studies almost never show study participants gaining muscle and losing fat simultaneously, unless they're sponsored by a supplement company, and even then the results tend to be tossed into the "too good to be true" junk pile.

But one study, published in 1983 in the now defunct *Canadian Journal of Applied Sport Science*s, really did show this effect. And given the reputation of the lead researcher, Michael Stone,** I'm confident the results weren't invented.

Here's what happened:

Stone and his colleagues took nine aspiring Olympic lifters and put them on an eight-week program.

The subjects' muscle mass increased by five pounds, on average, while body fat declined three percentage points. On top of that, aerobic power increased, while resting heart rate and blood pressure decreased. About the only favorable results they *didn't* get were whiter teeth and fresher breath. (And, who knows, maybe they did and the researchers didn't bother recording it.)

Stone is now the chief exercise physiologist for the U.S. Olympic committee in Colorado Springs. I contacted him there to ask for more details. He said the lifters were mostly new to the iron game, so their bodies hadn't yet made the sort of adaptations that would prevent a more experienced lifter from gaining muscle and losing fat at the same time. The routines were mostly done with fairly high repetitions (like Alwyn's Fat-Loss programs in Chapter 18). And the exercises that were specific to Olympic weight lifting—variations on the snatch and clean-and-jerk—are ones you won't see anyone performing at your local Gold's or Bally's. In most modern gyms, you're more likely to hear a Puccini opera on the sound system than you are to see an Olympic lift.

There is a way to get around this, and that's by combining an hour of strength training with an hour of endurance work in the same session. So instead of lifting and running six hours a week, spread over six training sessions, you do two-hour sessions three times a week.

This program has been used in multiple studies at the University of Wisconsin–Madison, and indeed, study subjects who lifted and rode stationary bikes three times a week saw the same strength and muscle growth as the ones who only lifted three times a week and the same increases in endurance as those who only rode stationary bikes.

All of which is a bit counterintuitive. It's hard to imagine that two-hour combined workouts would produce better results than one-hour workouts in which you focus on one type of exercise. But the results have been replicated in several studies, so I have to think this isn't just the physiological equivalent of an accounting trick.

Still, how useful is the model? I mean, the only way I could train for two hours a day, three times a week, is by cutting back on my writing and editing work, which would produce a significant interference effect on my income. I suspect you're in the same boat.

Meanwhile, lots of people enjoy working out six days a week, mixing endurance and strength exercise. But what's the point if you know the strategy is self-defeating?

You can probably do both successfully if you limit the intensity of one or the other. That is, if you're serious about training for a 10K or half-marathon, use the weight workouts for muscle maintenance rather than trying to get bigger and stronger. And if your main goal is strength and size, do shorter and easier endurance workouts to maintain your capacity.

RESOLVING THE CARDIO CONTROVERSY

There's one sure and easy way to start an argument, if you're the combative type: Go to a fitness-oriented website's message boards and either praise or condemn endurance exercise. You can bet you'll find plenty of disagreement from your fellow posters, no matter which position you take.

Alwyn has endured so many of these arguments that he would qualify for the Congressional Medal of Rhetorical Futility, if such a thing existed.

The problem, Alwyn has told me, is one of definition. "Cardio" and "aerobics" are used interchangeably, as synonyms for "endurance." In Alwyn's view, they shouldn't be. Here's how he defines them:

Cardio

This word should be used for any type of exercise that makes the heart and lungs work harder. Look back at "The Greatest Program Ever" on page 84. Guys in that study increased their aerobic power while also losing fat—exactly what you'd expect from "cardio" exercise. Except they accomplished this while doing Olympic-style weight lifting, which also increased their strength and muscle mass.

I've also heard about this effect from a friend training for a Strongman competition. The events generally take a couple minutes or less and are designed to test not only strength and power but also how long a competitor can continue a maximum effort. You don't have to compete to see how the events would force a contestant's heart and lungs to work full-out.

My friend told me that his VO_2 max, the scientific measure of aerobic power, increased dramatically during his Strongman training. This despite the fact he did no training that would meet the following description of "aerobic" exercise.

Aerobic

This describes exercise that uses the aerobic energy system, one of three ways your body has to generate energy. Here's what they are and how they work:

Phosphagen system: This energy system uses two substances—adenosine triphosphate (ATP) and creatine phosphate (CP)—for short, intense bursts of speed and power. Your body stores, at most, ten seconds' worth of ready-to-use ATP and CP.

Anaerobic glycolysis: Your body refuels itself by breaking down glycogen, the sugar in your muscles, and producing lactate as a by-product. The lactate can in turn be used for muscle fuel. The best-trained athletes in sports like boxing, wrestling, and intermediate-distance running (such as the 800-meter) can rely on their glycolytic energy system for up to two minutes. Mere mortals like us probably poop out in sixty seconds or less.

Aerobic metabolism: This is the easiest way for your body to generate energy for movement. You use it all the time, at rest or in motion. It uses oxygen ("aerobic" literally means "with oxygen") to burn a combination of fat and glycogen to produce energy.

Your body doesn't use just one system at a time. Let's say you're walking to the bus stop, using your aerobic energy system, and suddenly realize you'll miss the bus if you don't run the final two blocks. Energy for those first few steps will come from your phosphagen system, buying time for your glycolytic system to kick in. But that doesn't mean your aerobic system has shut down; it's simply adjusting to the new demands and will be back in play after about twenty to thirty seconds of running.

Thus, your run to the bus stop will involve all three energy systems.

Another example: downhill skiing. Your three energy systems—separately and together—will all be active in different parts of the run.

Conversely, in a basketball or football game, you'll hardly use your aerobic energy system at all, except when play is stopped. Hockey and soccer use a combination of

Metabolic Overdrive

Alwyn has a simple and brutally effective way to use your anaerobic energy systems for fat loss. He calls it "afterburn," meaning it burns some calories when you do it, and lots of calories afterward, via EPOC.

Here's how it works. The example given is for a stationary bike, but you can (and Alwyn says you should) try it in a variety of settings—running on a track or treadmill, swimming, riding a bike, rowing. You could even do it with calisthenic exercises, such as sit-ups, push-ups, lunges, or squats.

Warm-up: five minutes, very easy pace

Rounds: three minutes each. Crank up the tension as high as you can handle for sixty seconds. (Start conservatively; it's better to go to a higher tension for subsequent rounds than to blow your wad on this first one.) Then back off by riding at a moderate pace for two minutes.

Cool-down: five minutes, very easy pace

Sample sixteen-week plan; you perform these workouts on their own, or following a weight workout:

Weeks 1–4: Do 3 rounds, 3 times per week. Counting the warm-up and cool-down, this is a 19-minute workout.

Weeks 5–8: Do 4 rounds, 4 times a week. These are 22-minute workouts.

Weeks 9–12: Do 5 rounds, 4 times a week. These are 25-minute workouts.

Weeks 12–16: Do 6 rounds, 5 times a week. These are 28-minute workouts.

Alwyn says his clients typically lose a pound or two of fat per week while using this program. Actual results may vary, of course, but if you follow the nutrition guidelines in Part 5, while doing a strength-training routine three or four times a week, you should see fast and continuous fat loss.

the two anaerobic ("without oxygen") systems, along with aerobic metabolism. Baseball players have little use for the glycolytic or aerobic systems; most of the action is flat-out and takes just a few seconds, so almost all of it involves the phosphagen system. (Except the groin-scratching; that's purely aerobic.)

I go into all this detail to make this point:

There's nothing special about your aerobic energy system that needs to be trained. Your body already knows how and when to use it.

If you're pursuing a sport that uses the aerobic system—running, swimming, cycling, hockey, soccer—then of course you need to focus on developing the type of aerobic fitness that will help you succeed.

If you're so completely out of shape that you avoid going out on dates for fear you'll pass out during sex, then you need to build up some level of conditioning. A good benchmark is being able to walk or ride a bike for twenty minutes without an EMT escort.

But if you're in decent shape, and have no ambitions in sports involving the aerobic energy system, there's absolutely no reason for you to go out and run or ride long distances. Do it if you enjoy it. But if you don't like it and can't think of any particular reason to do it, don't.

Put another way: The captain has turned off the "aerobics" light. You're now free to move about the weight room.

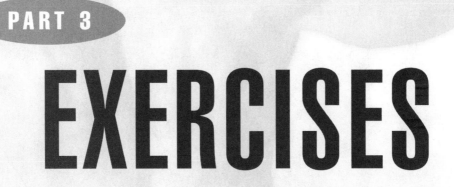

PART 3

EXERCISES

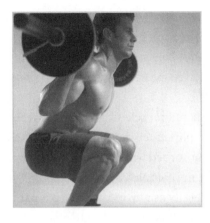

Squat

My FIRST EXPERIENCE with the squat wasn't a good one. I was in a gym in Anaheim, California, in 1984, doing my normal lower-body routine of leg presses, leg extensions, and leg curls. (Youth truly is wasted on the young.)

Somehow, I got talked into trying squats. I think this may have been the first gym I'd ever used that had an actual squat rack, so I figured, "What the hell." But instead of doing squats the way most guys do them, stopping well short of the point at which my thighs are parallel to the floor, these guys convinced me that the only way to squat was to do it all the way. Butt to calves.

So I tried it.

Once.

The next time I squatted was about twelve years later, and the experience was much better. As the newbie fitness editor of *Men's Fitness,* I assigned a workout feature to Bill Starr,* a legendary lifter and strength coach and a prolific author of articles about lifting.

He designed a strength- and power-based program, built around three key lifts:

squat, bench press, high pull. I started with just the forty-five-pound Olympic bar and focused on increasing my strength and range of motion gradually and carefully. If I were the type to be easily embarrassed—you've probably guessed by now that I'm not—I would've been ashamed for my coworkers to see me at the gym working my way up to using actual weight plates on the bar.

But, even with those starter weights, my strength and muscle size increased week after week. Several coworkers mentioned that my physique was thickening up (a compliment to a lifter). I hadn't noticed. I'd been so absorbed with learning these new exercises that one of the biggest benefits had caught me completely by surprise.

Today, I can sing the praises of the squat as earnestly as anyone. I never got particularly strong by lifelong-lifter standards; my personal record is a single repetition with 305 pounds at a body weight of about 185. Not bad, but not anything to include in the Christmas letter, either.

I now look forward to the squats in my workout programs as much as or more than any other exercise. Maybe I'm just weird, but I think there's something about a heavy bar on your shoulders that clears your mind of distractions and puts you in the moment.

THE MUSCLES

If you talk to Ian King, the Australian strength coach and my coauthor on *Book of Muscle,* you'll come away believing that the squat is a "quad dominant" exercise, meaning that the muscles most engaged are the quadriceps on the front of your thighs. Their primary function is to straighten your knee when it's bent.

If you talk to Louie Simmons, training guru to the world-class powerlifters at Westside Barbell in Columbus, Ohio, you'll come away believing that the quadriceps are the enemy of the successful squatter. Simmons believes the power behind the squat should come, literally, from behind—the gluteals and hamstrings.

Who's right?

Both, actually.

A joint USC-UCLA study published in 2003 looked at two different ways to squat, and the muscles involved in each. A traditional squat, the way we show it here, emphasizes action at the knee joint over hip movement.

But Simmons trains his powerlifters to squat a different way, using an exercise called a "box squat." They descend until they're sitting on a box (or bench, or chair). They pause on the box, then rise to the standing position. They can't sit down on a box in powerlifting competitions, but that's the way they train, setting the muscle-action patterns that they replicate in contests when they don't have the box. The study showed that this type of squat uses more hip action than the traditional squat and less knee and ankle movement. (The study used older adults as subjects, but I think it's safe to say the results accurately describe the divergent muscle-use philosophies of King and Simmons.)

One other tidbit about muscle action in the squat:

A 2001 study in *Medicine & Science in Sports & Exercise* showed that quadriceps involvement is greatest at the bottom of the movement, when the lifter is just starting his ascent back to the starting position. Hamstring involvement is greatest when the lifter is about one-third of the way to the top.

Why does that matter?

Many lifters short-change themselves on the squat by not descending all the way down to the point at which their upper thighs are parallel to the floor. You don't need to go lower than that (as I learned the hard way back in 1984, it's not a fun neighborhood to visit), but you should try to lower yourself to parallel, even though it means using lighter weights than you'd be able to handle if you stopped short.

FUNCTIONAL IMPORTANCE

Squats are used in workout programs for athletes in virtually every sport requiring lower-body strength and power, and with good reason: A 1997 study in the *Journal of Sports Science* showed that a training program involving heavy squats increased forty-meter sprint speed by 2.2 percent and six-second cycle performance (a measure of lower-body muscle power) by 9 percent.

For athletes who need to jump higher (basketball, volleyball, and football players, for example), the squat has been the mainstay exercise for decades.

TECHNIQUE

Back in Chapter 2, when I first described the squat, I asked you to imagine a time when your lower body was so weak you couldn't get up out of a chair in time to get to the bathroom.

Forget about urinating, but continue thinking about that chair:

If you were to lower yourself into a chair, how would you do it? The movement would start at the hip joint, with you pushing your butt backward toward the chair.

Your knees wouldn't bend until they had to, when your butt starts moving downward as well as backward.

Squatting works the same way.

No matter which variation you're doing, you lead the way with your butt, pushing your hips back; knee action will take care of itself.

If you watch someone at the gym with poor squat form, you'll probably see him bend his knees too soon, before his hips have moved back. Bending your knees so early does two things, both of them bad:

- Your knees will move forward, over your feet, which puts unnecessary strain on the knee joints.
- Your knees will probably buckle in a bit, which puts a different kind of strain on the connective tissues in your knees.

A third problem is that your heels may come up off the floor. This could be a separate issue, or a consequence of the knees bending too soon. Either way, it's bad for your balance—you want your weight over the middles of your feet, not over your toes—and it does your knees no favors.

A perfect descent ends with you sitting comfortably, with your upper thighs parallel to the floor, or even a bit below that point. There should be no strain anywhere—not on your knees, not on your hips, not on your lower back.

If someone were to take a snapshot of you from the side, perfect form would look like this:

- Your shoulders would be directly over the middles of your feet.
- Your torso and lower legs would probably be at the same angle to the floor—leaning forward slightly, but never dramatically.
- Your eyes would point forward, not up or down.
- Your knees could be over the middles of your feet . . . or farther forward, over your toes . . . or anywhere in between. Your individual biomechanics (including bone length and the degree of flexibility in your ankle joints) will determine where your knees go when the rest of your body is in the proper position. Some people will squat with their knees out past their toes and never have knee problems. But this I guarantee: If your knees end up to the inside of your feet—if your knees buckle inward, in other words—you're screwed. *That* will hurt your knees.

From that position, you rise, initiating the movement from your feet. Literally, you press your feet into the floor (always the middle of the feet, never the toes). As you rise, the knee joints should start to straighten before your hips. If your hips come up first, your torso will lean farther forward, and that's bad; it puts your lower back at much greater risk.

That's not to say the movement is powered entirely by your quadriceps down at the bottom. Yes, the muscle's working hardest down there, but your knees are protected by the simultaneous contraction of all the muscles that cross it, including the hamstrings and calf muscles.

The joints in your lower back should not move at all. You need to stiffen your midsection muscles, including those in your lower back, and keep them stiff throughout the exercise—while you're lowering, when you're paused at the bottom, and especially when you stand up.

What you will not do is suck in your abs, even though you see guys in body-

90 Degrees from Nowhere

Fitness and bodybuilding magazines have gotten the idea that the ideal knee angle in a squat is 90 degrees. Bend your knees more than 90 degrees, and they come apart. This kind of advice results in guys stopping their descent well before the point at which their upper thighs are parallel to the floor.

Not only are they limiting muscle growth by stopping short, they're probably putting their knees at greater risk of damage than if they descended lower.

The reason: 90 degrees is a notoriously weak angle for your knees, as physical therapist and strength coach Bill Hartman explained to me recently. As you descend lower than that point, your hamstrings and quadriceps work together to protect your knee joints.

That doesn't mean every guy can descend beyond 90 degrees safely; if you have past or current knee injuries, you'll have to figure out on your own (or with a trainer or physical therapist) the angles that work for you.

Assuming you're injury-free, the angle of your knees in the bottom position will vary greatly, depending on your biomechanics. If you're tall or just have exceptionally long legs, you may hit the parallel position with your knees close to 90 degrees. Guys with shorter leg bones will bend their knees much more to get down to parallel.

How low should you go, assuming no knee pain at any angle? Once again, it's all about your back. The lowest descent you can manage without changing the arch in your lower back and without any pain in your knees, hips, or back is the right one for you.

Hand Check

If you're confused about exactly when your lower back shifts out of its natural and proper alignment, have a friend give you a hand. Or a trainer, or training partner, or whoever you trust to put a palm across your lower back. Have him or her keep the hand in place as you descend, and tell you when your lower back moves. That's the lowest safe depth for you now.

If you have to stop before your upper thighs are parallel to the floor (and it's a good bet you will, if you've never squatted before), keep working at achieving that lower angle. You may need more flexibility in your hamstrings or hip flexors, but with practice you should improve your safe range of motion.

---

building magazines who seem to have done just that when squatting. (It's stupid to photograph guys squatting with their shirts off, but magazines do it all the time. As soon as the shirt comes off, the abs come in, whether it's appropriate for that exercise or not.) The squat is an ugly exercise. You end up with your belly pushed out slightly; that's how you form the protective belt for your spine.

THE EXERCISES

✳ Squat

USED IN: Break-In; Fat-Loss I and III; Hypertrophy I; Strength I, II, and III

SETUP: Place a barbell on the supports of the squat rack so that it's at upper-chest level. If the rack has safety rails on the sides, set them just below crotch level. (You want to be able to execute a deep squat without hitting those rails; they shouldn't come into play unless you get stuck on a maximum-effort squat, in which case you can simply slide the bar off your shoulders so it lands on the rails.) Duck under the bar and rest it across your upper traps, with your knees slightly bent. Grab the bar with a wide, overhand grip. Now lift it off the supports and step back so you can safely raise and lower the weights without hitting anything. (We didn't use a squat rack in these photos so we could give you a clearer view of the exercise form. You'll note that we use that strategy in several places in *New Rules of Lifting*. In Chapter 11, for example, we show barbell bench presses performed on a bench without uprights. In all these cases, we thought it would be more helpful for you to see the model perform the exercise without the equipment blocking his arms or legs.)

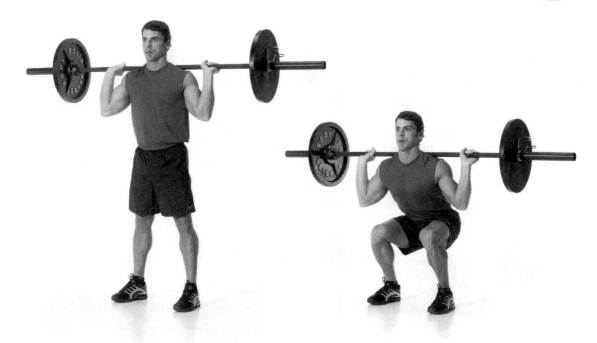

LOWERING: Stand with your feet shoulder-width apart, or just a bit wider, your toes pointed straight ahead or angled out slightly, your shoulders tight and eyes focused straight ahead. Push your hips back, as if sitting in a chair, and lower yourself until your upper thighs are parallel to the floor, or your back starts to lose its natural arch, whichever comes first.

LIFTING: Push down through the middles of your feet—never the toes—and stand straight up. You want your torso going up and straightening, not leaning farther forward.

FOR HYPERTROPHY AND FAT-LOSS PROGRAMS: When Alwyn trains clients for these goals, he doesn't allow them to straighten their knees fully at the top of the movement. When you get almost to the top of the movement, immediately reverse directions and lower yourself for the next rep. In Strength programs, however, you'll need to stop at the top and take a deep breath (if not two) before the next rep.

Variations

✳ Heels-raised back squat, one-and-a-quarter style

USED IN: Hypertrophy III

SAME AS ABOVE, EXCEPT . . . Set a pair of weight plates (5- or 10-pounders) on the floor behind you, and place your heels on the plates. Then lower yourself as described, but rise up just a quarter of the way. Lower yourself back down, then rise to the standing position. That's one repetition.

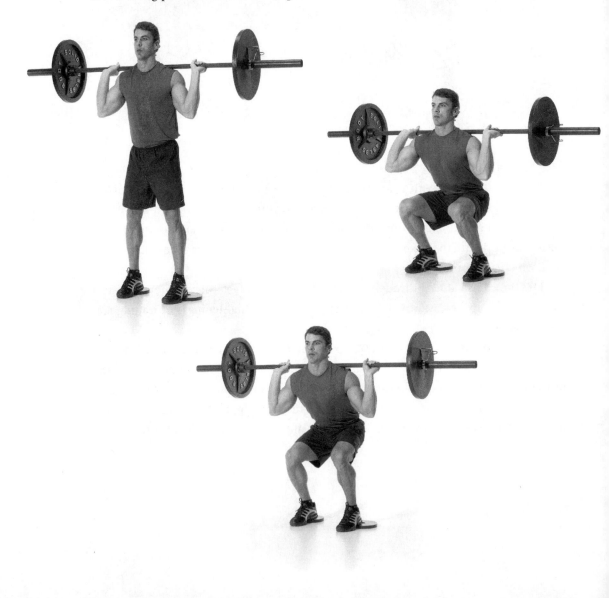

✴ Front squat

USED IN: Fat-Loss II and III

SAME AS ABOVE, EXCEPT . . . Instead of ducking under the bar, you're going to rest it on your front shoulders. Grab it with an overhand, shoulder-width grip, and rotate your arms upward until your upper arms are nearly parallel to the floor. This turns your front deltoids into a pair of hooks to hold the bar in place. You won't be able to grasp the bar with your hands in this position; instead, let it roll to the ends of your fingertips. As long as you keep your arms up, it'll stay in place.

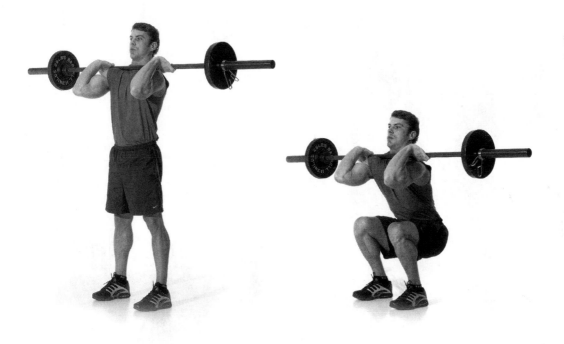

✴ Quarter squat

USED IN: Strength II and III

SAME AS ABOVE, EXCEPT . . . You're going to use weights heavier than you could squat to full range. So this time, you need to set up those side supports on the squat rack so they're about at the level of your upper hips. Go down just a quarter of the distance.

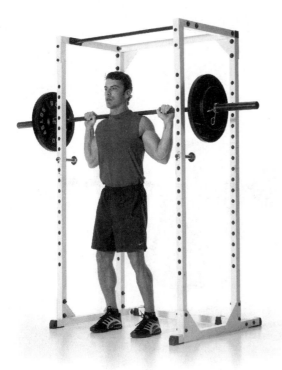

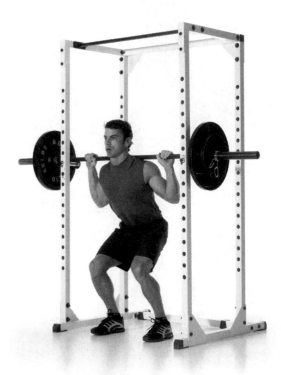

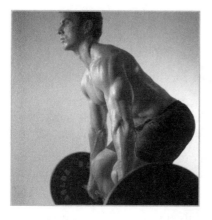

Deadlift

Back in Chapter 2, I described the deadlift as "perhaps the most useful exercise you can do with weights." Now here we are in Chapter 9, and I still agree with myself. (Funny how that works, especially the closer I get to my deadline.)

But proper form in the deadlift, unlike the squat, involves some counterintuitive movements. I don't mean that people in the gym just instinctively do squats with perfect form—nothing could be further from the truth.

Good form in the squat somewhat resembles sitting back in a chair—something we all know how to do—at least at the beginning of the movement. The deadlift, conversely, starts with a position that few people will assume without being taught. If there's something on the floor that needs to be picked up, your instinct, and mine, and everyone else's, is to bend forward at the waist and pick it up.

Even trained professionals would tell you that this movement is harmless if the object on the floor is essentially weightless. But in reality, even then it's not. Any type of uncalculated forward bending at the waist is dangerous.

Case in point: Have you ever heard of someone who says he "threw out" his back while bending to pick up a washcloth in the shower? The conventional wisdom is that the injury must've been caused by stress. That is, he was under a lot of pressure at work, or his marriage was crumbling, or there was something about that washcloth that really pissed him off that day.

That's not the way it works, according to Stuart McGill,** the spine-mechanics guru at the University of Waterloo in Ontario.

In his second book, *Ultimate Back Fitness and Performance,* McGill says that back injuries can occur any time your body suffers what he calls "motor-control errors." In layman's terms, a motor-control error occurs when one particular muscle doesn't do what your other muscles need and expect it to do. It's the physiological equivalent of trying to drive a car with a flat tire.

If you're doing a big-muscle, heavy-weight exercise like a deadlift, your muscles are probably awake and alert, which is why an experienced lifter is unlikely to hurt himself, even when he handles some pretty serious iron.

But that same lifter may hurt his back doing something completely innocuous, like bending over to pick up a piece of paper off the floor.

The cause, McGill writes, is a motor-control error. Some muscles may be alert and doing what they're supposed to do to protect the lifter's spine. But others may not have switched themselves on properly.

That's one type of error: Some muscles fire, but other don't, and the ensuing imbalance causes the firing muscles to pull the spine too hard in one direction. If everything's working, muscles on each side of the spine pull equally hard, and the spine stays where it's supposed to. If a muscle on one side fails to go into action, you could have an injury.

A second type of error occurs when the task seems so easy that none of the protective muscles fire. McGill cites research showing that it doesn't take much movement to damage "passive" muscles.

His own research has shown that even the strongest lifters can hurt themselves doing exercises they know how to do. All it takes is one motor-control error, one tiny muscle slacking off when all the others are pulling with every available fiber and neuron, and the lifter could hurt himself.

I guess I'm offering two lessons here:

1. No matter how simple the task, if your back is involved, pay attention to what you're doing.
2. On heavy lifts, focus is everything. The heavier the lift, the more extreme your focus needs to be.

Now, here's what I started to write about the deadlift:

You can't let your back, even for a second, slip out of natural shape, which includes a slight arch in the lumbar spine. If you try to lift with a rounded back—in other words, if you lose that arch—it's not a question of "if" you will hurt yourself. It's "when."

Which is not to say that proper deadlift form is difficult or tedious to learn. In fact, once you learn to lift barbells and dumbbells off the floor the correct way, you'll consciously lift everything with perfect form, whether it's a paper clip on the floor or a sofa you have to lug up three flights of stairs.

And your back will thank you for that.

THE MUSCLES

Your body has to use almost all its major muscles in a deadlift, with the exception of the chest. The prime movers are the "hip extensors"—the gluteals and hamstrings. The quadriceps get involved a bit—you start with your knees bent somewhat, and you have to straighten them to complete the lift—but this exercise works your butt and hamstrings more directly than any other.

Your lower back and midsection muscles have to stay tight, and even without moving they'll work like hell to keep your spine where it should be.

The other big player in the deadlift is your trapezius, which pulls your shoulder blades together in back.

But there's a lot more going on, especially when you start moving up to the heaviest possible weights. Your gripping muscles, of course, get a workout. But so do your biceps and triceps, which serve as the muscular link between your shoulders and shoulder blades and your forearms.

My friend Craig Ballantyne,* a strength coach in Toronto, once wrote something like this: Let's say you have two guys in a gym. One guy can deadlift a lot of weight, but never does biceps curls. The other guy can curl a lot of weight, but never does deadlifts. Odds are close to 100 percent that the first guy would also be able to curl a lot of weight, even though he never practices the exercise. But, Craig wrote, there's no guarantee the second guy could deadlift so much as a sack of cement off the ground. And even if he could, there's a chance he'd hurt himself doing it.

That, more than anything, describes the beauty of an ugly exercise like the deadlift. Learn this exercise, and you'll be able to lift just about anything. Avoid this exercise, and all bets are off.

FUNCTIONAL IMPORTANCE

Being able to lift something heavy off the ground, in my opinion, is its own reward. But it's also the key to most strength sports. The two Olympic lifts—snatch and clean-and-jerk—start with the barbell on the floor. The deadlift is the only one of the three events in powerlifting (the other two are the squat and bench press) in which the bar starts on the floor. It comes last in powerlifting contests, and competitors in that sport have this saying:

"The meet doesn't start until the bar hits the floor."

Translation: Someone who's particularly good at the bench press and squat may not be equally good at the deadlift. (Competitively, the deadlift is kind of a freakish move, in that it favors lifters with longer arms, who can use more leverage to get the bar off the floor; long arms are a distinct disadvantage in the bench press.) So a lifter who's leading his weight class after the first two events may very well get smoked in the deadlift and end up losing the first-place trophy to someone whose butt he just kicked in the bench and squat.

Few of this book's readers aspire to compete in strength sports, but I think there's a general point to extrapolate here: Back strength matters in every endeavor, whether we're talking about sports (virtually every athlete in the world is trained with the exercises shown on the following pages) or real life. The guy who can carry the beer keg up to the second-floor deck is always the most popular guy at the party (at least until the keg is tapped, and the rules of attraction kick in).

TECHNIQUE

As you may have noticed from the long, discursive story about blowing your back out while picking up a washcloth in the shower, the most important aspect of the deadlift is your lower-back position.

So let's start with that. Set an object on the floor so you can grab it just below your knees. A dumbbell, resting on one end so it's vertical on the floor, works well.

Now stand over it with your feet about shoulder-width apart, toes pointing forward. Push your hips back, as in the squat. This time, you're just trying to get low enough to allow yourself to grab the top of the dumbbell with your arms straight and your shoulders directly over the weight.

Your knees will be bent somewhat, but how much they're bent doesn't matter. What matters is the position of your back. You want your back to remain slightly

Going Against Type

Your body has two main types of muscle fibers: Type I fibers are also called "slow-twitch," meaning they're endurance-oriented. Type II fibers are also called "fast-twitch," meaning they handle everything from a baseball or golf swing lasting a second or two to a sprint that lasts twenty to thirty seconds. Most of us in the training biz assume that athletes who need strength and power to succeed will have a greater percentage of fast-twitch fibers.

But Andy Fry** and his colleagues at the University of Memphis showed otherwise. The researchers rounded up five competitive, drug-free powerlifters and compared them to five regular guys. The powerlifters averaged 224 pounds, the regular guys 187. (Average heights were the same—about five-foot-ten.)

The powerlifters were strong dudes, averaging best-ever lifts of 375 in the bench press and 625 in the deadlift. And they had no greater percentage of fast-twitch fibers than the non-lifters.

Yes, their fibers were bigger, and there were major differences in the subtypes of Type II fibers, which aren't worth describing here. The key is that guys who were very, very good at lifting heavy stuff had the same percentage of strength- and endurance-oriented muscle fibers as a random sample of non-lifters.

arched, although if you were doing this with your shirt off, your back would appear perfectly flat from your hips to the top of your neck.

That's because the muscles in your lower back will contract, obscuring the true angle of your spine. It doesn't matter. The real key is that you feel your lower back remain in the same position throughout the movement. (The hand-on-the-lower-back test I described in Chapter 8 works even better for deadlifts.)

Okay, so you've got your hands around the top of the dumbbell, your hips are back, your arms are straight, your shoulders are directly over the weight, and your eyes are pointed straight ahead.

All you need to do is lift, right?

Almost. First you need to tighten everything up—pull your shoulder blades together in back as much as possible, straighten your knees as much as you can, clench your midsection. (Just tighten it; don't suck it in.)

Now you're ready to lift.

Push down with your feet, as you did in the squat, and start the movement by straightening your knees. When the top of the weight is just past your knees, thrust your hips forward until you're standing up straight.

Then lower the weight along the same path, although you don't have to worry about doing it in the same sequence. Just keep the muscles in your middle body tight until the weight reaches the floor. Relax, then set up for the next repetition.

Remember to keep the "dead" in deadlift. That means each lift starts with the weight resting on the floor.

THE EXERCISES

✳ Deadlift

USED IN: Break-In; Fat-Loss I and III; Strength I, II, and III

SETUP: Load an Olympic barbell and set it on the floor. Squat over it with your feet about shoulder-width apart and toes pointed forward. Grab it with an overhand grip, your hands just outside your legs and your arms straight. Now roll the bar toward you until it's directly under your shoulders. Some guys start with the bar at their shins; others like the bar farther out, meaning they start with less of a bend in their knees. Both techniques are fine, as long as your lower back is slightly arched. Finally, tighten up everything, from your grip to your shoulders and on down to your feet.

LIFTING: Push straight down through the middles of your feet as you straighten your knees. Depending on your starting position, you'll either pull the bar to your

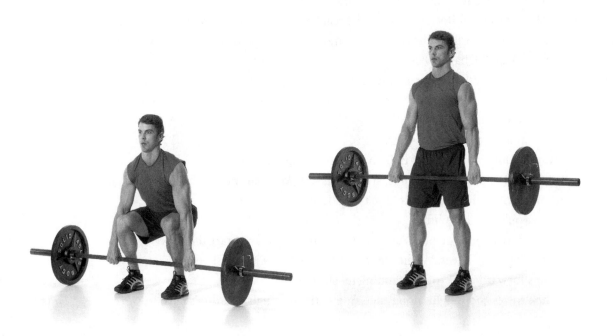

lower legs and then up, or straight up. Either way, the bar must stay in contact with your legs all the way up. With the bar past your knees, push your hips forward as you squeeze your shoulder blades together in back. This straightens your torso and squares your shoulders to complete the lift.

LOWERING: Lower the bar along your body to the floor. With heavy weights, you want to wear sweatpants when you deadlift. Otherwise, expect some scrapes on your shins.

MIXED GRIP: With your heaviest lifts, you'll need to switch to the mixed grip—one hand over and one hand under the bar. This takes a bit of getting used to, since at first it'll feel as if you're applying uneven torque to your spine. But in reality, the muscles that rotate your arm outward for the underhand grip—the rear deltoid and two small rotator-cuff muscles—have nothing to do with your spinal stability. The arm with the overhand grip will be slightly forward of the one with the underhand grip, which is why it feels as if it's twisting your spine. Your muscles, however, have to fire evenly on both sides of your spine, making it perfectly safe for experienced lifters doing Alwyn's Strength programs.

Variations

✳ Snatch-grip deadlift

USED IN: Fat-Loss II; Hypertrophy II

SAME AS ABOVE, EXCEPT . . . Take a wide grip, with your thumbs on the ring in the Olympic bar. You should feel the difference in your traps—they have to work harder to hold your shoulder blades in place with your arms out wide—and perhaps in your torso, just because it's a bit harder to control your balance.

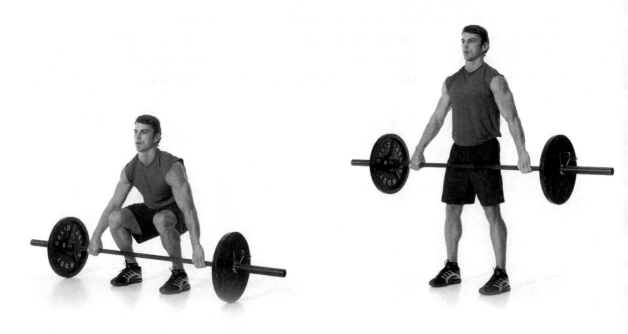

✳ Deadlift off box

USED IN: Fat-Loss III

SAME AS ABOVE, EXCEPT . . . Get a solid platform that's about four to six inches high. A step from the aerobics studio works well. You're going to stand on the box, and then do everything as described for the deadlift. Since the bar's lower, you'll have to start the lift with your body lower (and use less weight, of course). The extra challenge of that will help make regular deadlifts seem easier.

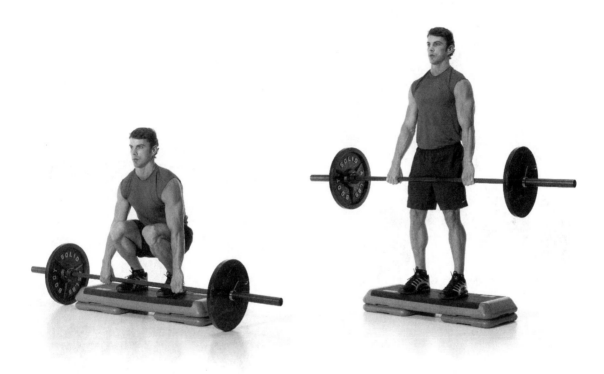

✳ Snatch-grip deadlift off box *(not shown)*

USED IN: Strength III

SAME AS ABOVE, EXCEPT . . . Stand on the box and take the wide grip described previously.

✳ Rack deadlift

USED IN: Strength II and III

SAME AS ABOVE, EXCEPT . . .   You're going to start with the bar resting on supports in the squat rack, just below knee level. This limited range of motion allows you to use much heavier weights.

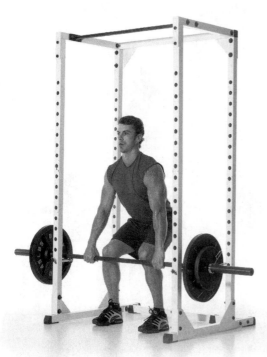

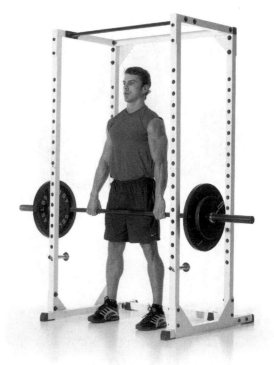

✳ Romanian deadlift

USED IN: Fat-Loss I; Strength I

SETUP: Load a barbell and hold it with an overhand grip that's just outside shoulder width. Stand with your arms straight and the bar in front of your thighs; your lower back is in its natural arch and your shoulders are pulled back. (It's the finishing position for the deadlift.)

LOWERING: Lower the bar along your thighs until it's just below your knees. Your hips will go back and your knees will bend a bit. The key is to keep your lower back in the same arch throughout.

LIFTING: Push your hips forward as you straighten your torso and pull the bar straight up along your thighs.

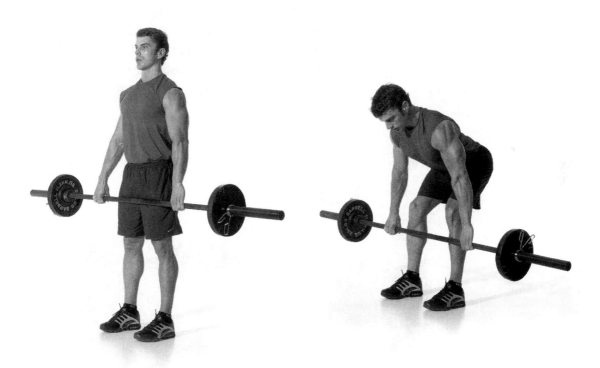

✳ Romanian deadlift/row

See Chapter 14.

✳ Good morning

USED IN: Strength I and II

SETUP: Set up a lightly loaded barbell in the rack, at the same height you'd use for squats. (You probably want to start with just the bar if you've never done this before.) Set it on your traps, lift it off the supports, and step back. You want your feet positioned and your posture set as described for the squat in Chapter 8.

LOWERING: Push your hips back as you bend your torso forward. The farther you bend forward, the more your knees will bend, which is fine—do what your body wants to do. The key is to keep your lower back in its natural arch throughout. Never compromise that arch for the sake of a deeper range of motion. The second key is to keep your head and neck in the same posture. That means you'll be looking down at the floor at the bottom of the movement. Most guys will try to keep their eyes up to watch themselves in the mirror, but that distorts your posture and limits your strength.

LIFTING: Push your hips forward as you rise to the starting position. Remember, it's all in the hips, meaning the entire focus here is on your gluteals and hamstrings, which move your hips forward. If you feel yourself using your knees to generate momentum, stop the set. At that point, you're just doing squats with light weights and bad form.

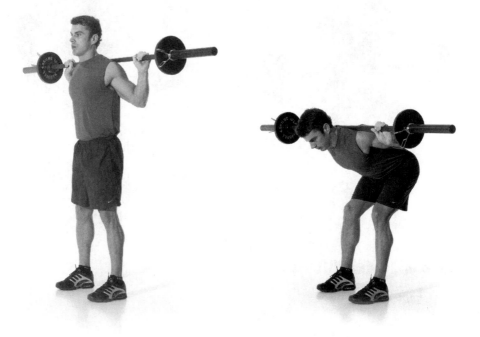

Variation

✳ Zercher good morning

USED IN: Strength III

SAME AS ABOVE, EXCEPT . . . You'll hold the bar in front of you, in the crook of your arms, instead of across your back. Make sure you wrap a towel around the bar, or use one of those pads some lifters put on the bar when they do squats. Or at least wear a long-sleeved sweatshirt when you do the lift. Otherwise, the bar will leave some ugly red trails on your biceps and forearms.

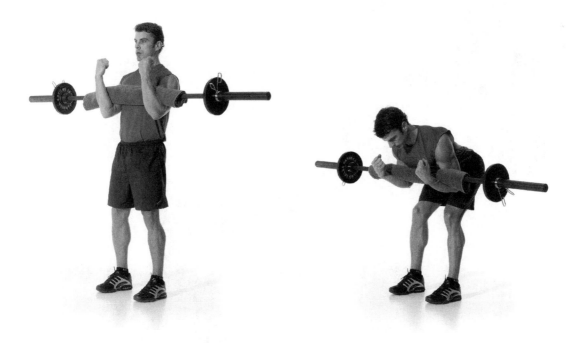

✳ Seated good morning

USED IN: Strength III

SAME AS ABOVE, EXCEPT . . . You'll do it seated on the end of a bench. The range of motion is shorter, but it really, *really* forces you to focus on keeping your lower back in its proper arch.

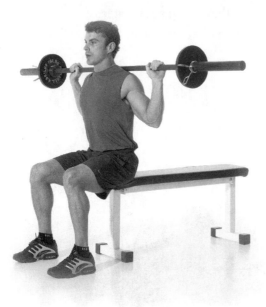

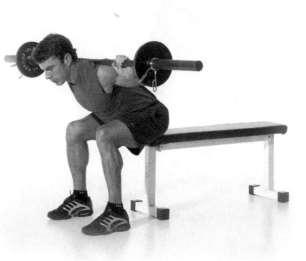

✳ Split good morning

See Chapter 14.

✳ Supine hip extension

USED IN: Fat-Loss I

SETUP: Grab a Swiss ball and lie on your back on the floor with your heels and lower legs on the ball, your legs straight, and your arms straight out to your sides.

LIFTING: Using your gluteals and hamstrings, push your hips up so your body forms a straight line from your ankles to your shoulders.

LOWERING: Bring your hips down but don't allow them to touch the floor again until you've done all the repetitions. You want to keep some tension on your rear-body muscles.

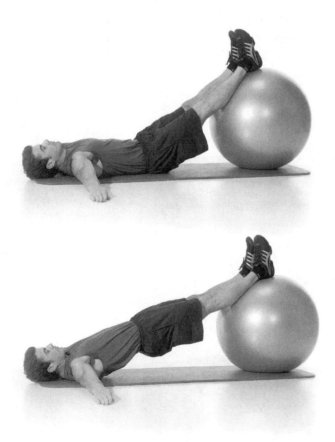

Variation

✳ Supine hip extension with leg curl

USED IN: Fat-Loss II

SAME AS ABOVE, EXCEPT . . . When your body is in that straight line, use your hamstrings to pull the ball toward you until your feet are flat on the ball, your knees are bent about 90 degrees, and your body forms a straight line from your knees to your shoulders. You should feel it in your calves as well as your hamstrings, since your calves assist on the leg curl. (Bet you didn't know that!) The movement is doubly challenging to your hamstrings, which aren't used to exerting force in two directions at once: They're helping your gluteals keep your body straight—a movement called "hip extension"—and also forcefully bending your knees, which is called "knee flexion." Once you try these, you'll never go back to leg curls on the sissy machines.

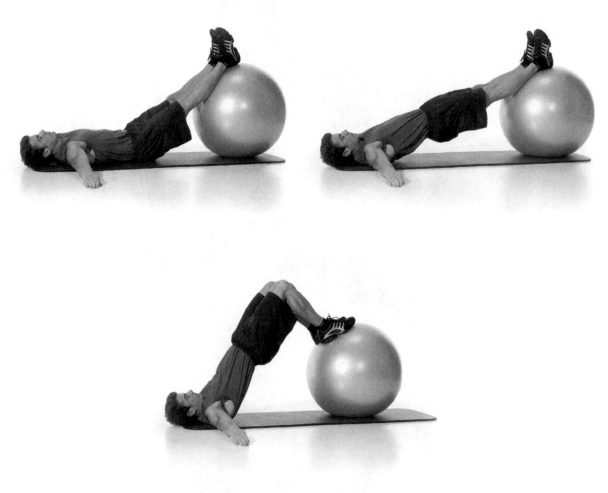

✳ Back extension

USED IN: Strength I and II

SET-UP: Position yourself on the back-extension apparatus (Roman chair) so your heels are under the rear pads and your hips are across the main pads. Your body should form a straight line from your ankles to your neck. You can hold your hands across your chest (that's the easiest position), up next to your ears, or straight out to the sides or in front of you (hardest). If you can easily do all the designated reps in the hardest position, hold a weight plate across your chest with your hands.

LOWERING: Bend at the hips (not at the waist), folding your body like a jackknife.

LIFTING: Pull your body back up to the starting position, using your gluteals and hamstrings. If you notice women congregating nearby when you do back extensions, you're doing them right.

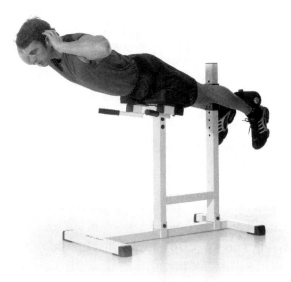

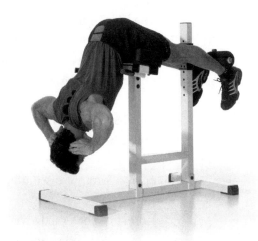

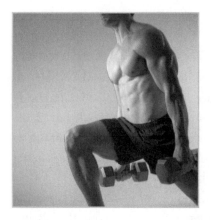

Lunge

THERE WAS A TIME when my knees hurt just thinking about lunges. I'd started playing basketball at age thirty-six, and by the time I hit my mid-forties, my knees were wrecked.

The irony is that just when I finally learned what I was supposed to be doing on the court—how to move without the ball, how to dribble and shoot layups with either hand, how to play better defense—my knees were so battered that I couldn't do any of the things I was learning. I found myself unable to run or jump, and basketball isn't a good recreational choice for floor-bound walkers.

And, back to the point of this chapter, I couldn't even think about doing exercises like lunges in the gym.

Now, two years after hanging up my basketball shoes, I can do all the exercises in this chapter without discomfort. I also incorporate lunges into my warm-ups before most workouts.

I use my not-exactly-tragic basketball story to illustrate an important point about knee pain and strength-training exercises:

If your knees are already injured from something else, exercises like squats and lunges will hurt more than they would if you were doing them with pain-free hinges. And people who already have knee pain are more likely to struggle to perform exercises correctly, as shown in an Australian study published in 2002 in the *Journal of Orthopedic Research.* The researchers couldn't determine if knee pain caused the loss of knee-joint coordination or if poor coordination caused the pain. A follow-up study, published in the same journal in 2005, tried to answer the question by inducing pain in subjects with healthy knees. (They injected saline beneath the kneecaps to create swelling and pressure. Ouch!) The induced pain didn't cause a loss of coordination, which suggests that perhaps faulty movement patterns predispose someone to knee pain. In other words, the chicken precedes the egg.

That brings up this question: When we're talking about an exercise like the lunge, what would "poor knee-joint coordination" look like? The simplest answer is one of the standards of magazine articles and books about lifting: The knee should never extend past the toes on a lunge.

But is that knees-past-toes position really injurious? Good luck finding an answer. I couldn't find anything definitive, mostly because the real answer seems to be "it depends." Alwyn notes that the knees go out past the toes all the time in sports and real-life situations. (Walking up stairs, for example.) He believes, after a lifetime as a high-level athlete and trainer of high-level athletes, that there's no real harm in the knees going forward. Yes, it certainly places the knees under more pressure; you have the biggest bones on your body, the thighbones, pushing forward on the kneecaps. But since the stress happens in a controlled situation when you're lifting, it's like any other exercise-induced challenge to your muscles, bones, and connective tissues. You're teaching your knees to be stronger in that position, and you're doing so in a systematic way, using heavier weights as you get stronger and more skilled at the exercise.

That doesn't mean the weight itself should be out over your knees. On the lunge or squat, you want the barbells or dumbbells directly over your heels or the middle of your feet. And it makes sense to work toward squatting or lunging with your lower legs more vertical than diagonal.

But some lifters, because of the length of their bones in relation to each other, or the relative stiffness or flexibility of their ankle and hip joints, won't be able to squat or lunge with the recommended lower-leg verticality.

And they'll probably do fine with their knees farther forward, as long as they lift through a pain-free range of motion. (If it hurts, no matter how vertical your shins may be, you need to make adjustments until you can lift without pain.)

The mistake that's most likely to hurt your knees, and one that you see every day in every gym, is allowing your knees to drift inward or (more rarely) outward during a squat or lunge. The knees should point toward the second toe on the way up and the way down. Deviating from that path, especially when using heavy weights, can pull the kneecap out of its path. (Physiological side note: The kneecap is just a small hunk of bone held in place by the muscles, cartilage, tendons, and ligaments surrounding the knee joint.) Another problem is that the knees' collateral ligaments—medial (MCL) and lateral (LCL)—can get overstretched and thus weakened by the bad-form, heavy-weights combo.

When you squat with proper form, keeping the knees aligned with the toes, your knees have a complex protective system, including some of your body's strongest muscles—the quadriceps, hamstrings, and calves. But when that knee rolls in or out, there's little to protect it beyond those ligaments and pure, dumb luck.

THE MUSCLES

As with the squat and deadlift, virtually all lower-body muscles get into a lunge. The quadriceps straighten your knee when it's bent, and the hamstrings and gluteals straighten your hip when you return to the standing position.

However, because your legs are split apart, you're presenting an interesting and different challenge to the muscles on the inner and outer regions of your hips and thighs.

We know no real man would be caught dead on the adduction and abduction machines. (The first one trains inner-thigh muscles by forcing you to close your thighs against resistance, while the second works the outer hips and thighs by forcing you to spread 'em.)

If you look at an anatomical chart, though, you may wonder about those muscles. The inner-thigh muscles, for example, are actually pretty big, and have testosterone-friendly names like "adductor magnus." Who wouldn't want to develop his magnus? The outer-hip muscles look pretty cool, too. The gluteus medius, in particular, helps form the dimple surrounding the hip joint, and I think it's safe to say women like to see the dimple on a naked man. (No, I haven't done a survey; my scientific curiosity only goes so far.)

Women, of course, have no hesitation about training those muscles directly on the adductor and abductor machines. I suspect a lot of guys wonder if it's necessary. It's not. (Confess: You're relieved to know that, aren't you?)

Quick lesson in biomechanics: How important is opening or closing your legs in sports or real-life movements? Not very, right? So why does your body assign relatively big, strong muscles to those movements? Did our evolutionary path prepare us for Nautilus machines and interpretive dance?

Actually, the muscles are there mostly to provide stability: to prevent unwanted inward and outward movement of your hips. You can test this yourself by working up to heavy weights on lunges and wide-stance squats. Those muscles will grow. There's a reason advanced, steroid-using bodybuilders get chafed inner thighs.

A forward lunge offers a particular challenge to the outer-hip muscles, which have to work hard to keep you balanced. A step-up—a vertical lunge—forces your inner-thigh muscles to reconsider their purpose in life. The higher the step, the harder they'll work.

FUNCTIONAL IMPORTANCE

Picture a pitcher, the baseball kind. The power behind his pitches begins with his first movement toward the plate, a lunge. That's followed by a twist as his torso comes around toward the hitter. The last movement, a push, is what we consider a "throw" or "pitch."

A Little Leaguer could connect with a Randy Johnson fastball if it weren't for the lunge and twist that come before the pushing movement.

And, conversely, if you took the lunge and twist away from a hitter, all the steroids in the world wouldn't allow him to smack anything more dangerous than a lazy fly to shallow center.

In other words, in sports, the lunge is often the movement that powers our bodies to do the things we don't think of as lunges.

In real life, you often use the lunging movement in relative isolation—striding over the oil slick your "quality pre-owned vehicle" left in your garage; taking the stairs two at a time—but in sports, the lunge is almost always part of a complex series of movements.

A rock climber, for example, combines lunges with twists and pulls; a volleyball player combines lunges with twists and pushes. A wrestler will lunge, twist, and pull his opponent to the mat. A boxer will lunge, twist, and push a punch toward an opponent's jaw.

TECHNIQUE

A lunge can go in any direction—forward, sideways, backward, and every point in between. Many strength coaches and physical therapists work their athletes and clients through all 360 degrees of possibilities.

For our discussion, though, let's stick with the forward type.

You can do these as static lunges, in which you take a step forward with your left leg, say, then lower yourself until your right knee nearly touches the floor. Instead of stepping back to the original position, with your feet together, you do all your repetitions in that split position, then switch legs and repeat the set with your right leg forward.

In a dynamic lunge, you step forward and back on each repetition, usually alternating legs.

Another variation is the walking lunge, which Alwyn doesn't use in these programs. Instead of lunging forward and then stepping back, you continue taking lunge-steps forward.

We also include the step-up with the lunging exercises. Many trainers include step-ups with deadlift variations, since the step-up challenges the glutes and hamstrings much more than the quadriceps. But I think it's more similar to the lunge, as

Who Knees This?

Knees can blow up for all sorts of reasons. Some people, for example, are just screwed with a genetic predisposition to knee injuries or arthritis. Aging also is brutal to knees, as blood flow to the joints decreases and the connective tissues become weaker and less pliable. And on an athletic court or field, any kind of crazy thing can happen. All it takes is for one foot to zig when the rest of you zags, and that's it for one or more ligaments. A large study of Australian rugby players found that dry fields were a major cause of knee injuries. Players can execute sharper cuts on a dry field, putting them at greater risk for twisting and contact injuries. Wet fields mean it's harder to plant a foot and cut to the left or right, and it means your foot has less connection to the ground if someone plows into you. A good downpour should eliminate the risk of knee injuries altogether.

Your best defense against knee injury is simple: Warm up.

A 2002 study in the *British Journal of Sports Medicine* found that your "joint position appreciation"—coordination, in other words—increases when you warm up. The warm-up in this study was just four minutes long and included jogging and stretching.

Surely you can find four minutes to keep your knees safe.

a movement pattern, because you're forcing the muscles of one leg to do disproportionate work on each repetition. (Also, speaking as a chronic knee-acher, I think the step-up is the perfect lunge variation for guys who feel discomfort in the knee joint when doing conventional lunges.)

No matter the version you're doing, good form is what I described above: You want your knee aligned with your middle toe, and you generally want your lower leg as close to vertical as possible, with your knee joint bent at least 90 degrees.

THE EXERCISES

✳ Static lunge

USED IN: Break-In; Strength I

SET-UP: Set a barbell on the supports of a squat rack. Set the barbell on your trapezius with your shoulder blades pulled together. Step away from the supports and take a "split" stance, with your front heel about three feet in front of your rear toe. (If you're right-handed, start with your left leg out in front; as a general rule, always work your weaker or non-dominant side first.)

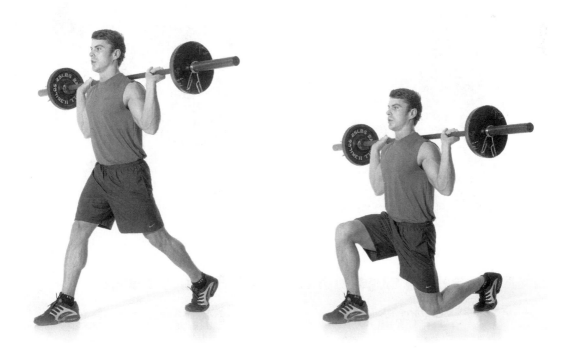

LOWERING: Lower your body so your front knee is bent about 90 degrees and your rear knee nearly touches the floor. Keep your torso as upright as possible.

LIFTING: Rise back to the split position. Finish all the reps, then switch legs and repeat the set.

Variations

✳ Dynamic lunge

USED IN: Fat-Loss II; Hypertrophy II; Strength II

SAME AS ABOVE, EXCEPT . . . You'll start with your feet parallel and hip-width apart, and lunge out and back, alternating legs on each repetition.

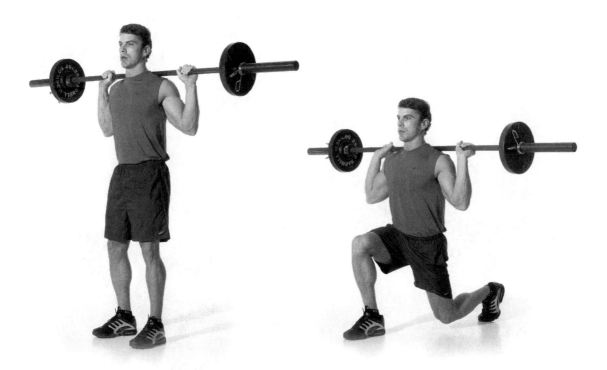

✳ Walking lunge with side bend, Rotational lunge

See Chapter 14.

✳ Bulgarian split squat

USED IN: Fat-Loss I and III; Hypertrophy I; Strength I and II

SETUP: Stand with your legs split, the top of your rear foot resting on a bench. (Again, start with your weaker leg, probably your left, in front.) Hold the dumbbells with straight arms, your palms facing your sides.

LOWERING: Lower your body until your front knee is bent about 90 degrees, while keeping your torso upright.

LIFTING: Rise back to the starting position. Do all your reps, then switch legs and repeat.

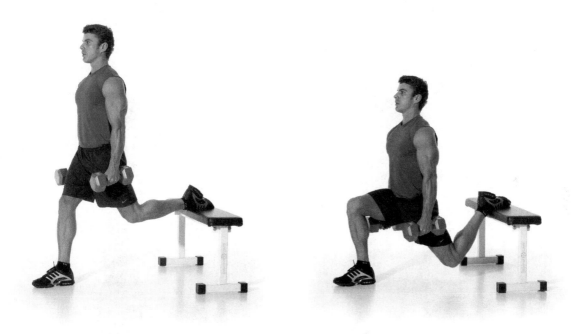

Variations

✳ Bulgarian split deadlift,
Bulgarian split squat with overhead press

See Chapter 14.

✳ Step-up

USED IN: Break-In; Fat-Loss III; Hypertrophy I and II; Strength I

SET-UP: Set up a box or stack of steps from the aerobics studio so that it's about knee-high. You can start lower (as shown in these photos) if you're a beginner, or go higher if you're advanced. Hold a pair of dumbbells at your sides.

LIFTING: Place your right foot flat on the step. Push down through your right foot to straighten your right leg and lift your entire body up. (Don't push off with your left leg; it's just along for the ride.) Set your left foot down on the step.

LOWERING: Step off with your left foot. As soon as it brushes the floor, lift again with your right leg. Finish all your reps, then switch legs and repeat the set.

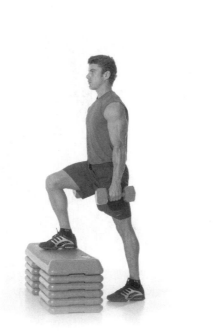 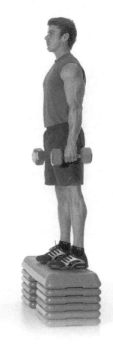

Variation

Although it's not specified in these workouts, you can hit your body with a bigger endurance challenge on the higher-rep sets by alternating legs on each rep. You start with both feet on the floor, step up with your left, lift your body, and touch your right foot to the step. Step down with your right, followed by your left. Then step up with your right, and touch your left foot on the step. Step down with your left, followed by your right. That's one repetition. I get dizzy trying to keep it straight—oxygen to the brain isn't a priority on high-rep step-ups—but if you want to try it, it's your option.

Barbell or Dumbbells?

On most exercises, there's a compelling reason why Alwyn chooses one or the other in any particular program. On lunges . . . well, it's not so compelling. Most of these lunges, split squats, and step-ups can be done just as effectively with barbells or dumbbells. A few guidelines:

1. If it's six-of-one, half-dozen-of-the-other, choose whichever is most convenient to use.

2. You can shake up your workouts by switching from barbell to dumbbells and back again from one workout to the next.

3. A barbell is awkward to use on Bulgarian split squats (and their many variations), walking lunges, and any type of angled lunge. You'll probably want to stick with dumbbells on these.

4. Conversely, switching from dumbbells to a barbell on the step-up makes it a different, almost supercharged exercise, since you've shifted the center of gravity upward. It's not for beginners or the timid, but in my experience, the barbell step-up rises above all other lunge variations as a lower-body muscle builder. And it's a great exercise for sharpening your focus in the gym; if you let your mind wander over to the bodies in the yoga studio with a heavy barbell on your shoulders . . . well, you don't really want to contemplate the many possible consequences of that strategy.

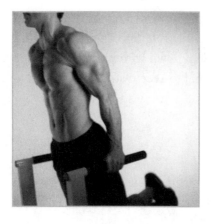

Push

I HAVE TO GET THIS off my chest:

I've been lifting weights almost three-quarters of my life. And I've never been able to bench-press worth a damn. My best-ever bench was 260 pounds, at a body weight of, I'd guess, 185 pounds. And I can't lift anything close to that now.

Excuses? I have a few. The bench press has never been a natural lift for me. My arms are too long and my torso too thin to offer any sort of biomechanical advantage. If I have a strength gene, it seems to have skipped a generation; I was always among the weakest boys in my peer group, until I started lifting weights at thirteen. (And even then, at best, I brought myself up to the median.) And sometime in my late teens, I smacked my sternum so hard in a sledding mishap (caught air going over an icy ridge, landed chest-first, smashed the wooden sled to smithereens, and possibly cracked my breastbone) that I was unable to do any heavy chest exercises without pain until my mid-twenties.

Still . . .

When I started lifting seriously heavy weights in my forties, I worked harder at the bench press than at any other lift. (As does almost every lifter.) And I still never got particularly good at it.

It shouldn't bother me. New Rule #6 tells me that the weight I lift is a tool to reach goals, not a goal in itself. And it's worth noting that I *wrote* New Rule #6.

So why do I care?

The short answer is because the bench press is the default exercise in modern gym culture—it's the one we all do, and the one most of us, at some point, have "maxed out" on. Thus, almost every meathead, mook, and gym rat in every American health club has a pretty good idea of how much he can bench. Whether he's doing it subtly or obnoxiously, you know almost every guy in the gym is measuring himself against you every time you load a barbell in the bench-press station.

An interesting question:

How did the bench press become the default exercise? It wasn't particularly popular until after World War II and seems to have gained its biggest momentum in the mid-1950s, when a Canadian Olympic weight lifter attributed his massive upper body to the bench press. Joe Weider, the bodybuilding guru, also pushed it in his magazines of that era. A 1957 article in *Muscle Power* magazine—one of the forerunners of *Muscle & Fitness*—declared the bench press "The Greatest Exercise of Them All." This provoked howls of derision from the editors of rival muscle magazines, who disdained bodybuilding in general and Weider in particular.

When I started lifting, around 1970, the bench press was an afterthought. The standing military press was regarded as the true test of strength, since few of us had benches in the makeshift gyms in our basements and carports.

But with the rise of health clubs and organized strength programs for professional and college sports teams, the bench press became the king of the weight room. *Pure Power* magazine suggested four reasons why:

1. It's easy to learn and practice.
2. Beginners make quick gains.
3. It works muscles you can see in the mirror.
4. It's a legitimate, contested lift in the sport of powerlifting.

I think that's a good list, and I'd add just one elaboration: When you do a bench press, it's easy to figure out if you completed the lift or not. If you lower the barbell until it touches your chest and then lift it until your elbows are straight ("lockout"), it's good. Some guys will still cheat by lifting their buttocks off the bench or claiming a completed lift even though a spotter helped them. This class of lifter regards it as a done deal, as long as the spotter shouts "All you!" while he's helping you finish the lift. (I'll say more about spotting in Chapter 20.)

Contrast that with an exercise like the squat, in which there's no real health-club standard for what constitutes a legitimately completed repetition. I've seen guys strut around like King Kong after a squat with such a short range of motion that their knees barely bent and straightened. Most gym rats, I think, would be shocked to learn that a squat doesn't count in a powerlifting competition unless the lifter's thighs "break parallel." That means the crease where his thigh meets his torso has to be lower than his knee. If you ever see anyone squat that low in a health club, take a picture, because it's a rare sight indeed.

And, while the deadlift is the least ambiguous of all the powerlifts—you either lift it off the floor or you don't—it's even more rarely seen in health clubs than the below-parallel squat.

So that brings me back to my dilemma: How do I stop caring so much about an exercise at which I'll never be very good?

Here's my four-step program. (I would've made it twelve steps, but that just sounds too hard.)

1. The bench press, functionally, isn't a very important lift—certainly not any more important than any other pushing exercise. In real life, there's really no equivalent of lying on your back and pushing a heavy thing off your chest with both arms moving at exactly the same angle and speed. Therefore, I'll force myself to do a variety of pushing exercises, at a variety of angles, using dumbbells as well as the barbell.

2. There's no reason to do the bench press first every time I use it in a workout. Yes, doing it first guarantees I'll perform better in that lift than any other in the program. But it also means I'll care about it more than any other. So, until I break my bench-press addiction, I'll make sure I do other lifts first, and use them to fulfill New Rule #5 ("The goal of each workout is to set a record"). That way I'll never have to worry about breaking my personal records in the bench press.

3. I will not watch other guys bench-press and compare myself to them. Unless their form is really bad, in which case I'll allow myself to feel smug and superior, but for reasons unrelated to pure strength.

4. I will not, under any circumstances, ask anyone how much he can bench. And if I think anyone is measuring himself against me, here's what I'll do: I'll load a bar with

405 pounds, then go to the bathroom. I'll come back ten minutes later, write down a number in my training log, and strip the weight off the bar. Unless the other guy has been watching the station nonstop for the entire ten minutes, he'll have no idea if I actually lifted the weight or not, and not knowing will drive him nuts.

THE MUSCLES

So far, I've used all my words in this chapter on the bench press, even though a pushing exercise can be anything from a shoulder press to a dip, with the bench press somewhere in the middle.

They all use the same muscles, with some variations based on particular regions of individual muscle groups.

Let's start with the chest: Its biggest muscle, the clam-shaped pectoralis major, has upper (clavicular) and middle (sternocostal) portions. There's also a lower part of the pectoralis, which is mildly interesting because its fibers originate from connective tissue at the top of the abdominal muscles. Functionally, it works along with the other portions of the muscle.

Every bodybuilder can tell you that if you want to hit the upper chest, you do presses on an inclined bench (which puts your shoulders higher than your hips). And if you want to hit that lower portion, the part that attaches to the abdominals, you do presses on a declined bench, so your shoulders are lower than your hips.

A 1995 study in the *Journal of Strength and Conditioning Research* challenged this belief. Turns out, the way to activate the upper chest is to use a narrow grip, with your thumbs twelve to eighteen inches apart. And a decline press didn't work the lower chest any harder than a flat-bench press.

Maybe all this matters for a serious bodybuilder. Regular gym rats? I'd be surprised if anyone could prove that a steady routine of, say, incline or decline bench presses would produce results measurably different from those obtained from using heavy weights on a flat bench.

I do strongly believe in changing angles and grip width throughout a program, but it's not because of my concern for some fibers an inch or two north of some other fibers. It's to give your shoulders a break. Constant pressing at the same angle, month after month and year after year, will probably wear down the connective tissues in your shoulder joints as quickly as it builds the muscles surrounding those joints.

I think it's very helpful to a long-haul lifter to think of muscles in terms of the joints they're responsible for moving. And almost all the "push" muscles work on the shoulder joint. Technically, I should add, there's more than one shoulder joint; I'm referring here to the "glenohumeral joint," the ball-and-socket junction where the top of the arm bone rolls around in a groove at the edge of the scapula.

Bodybuilders regard their "shoulders" as physiologically separate from their "pecs," but in reality the difference is one of surprisingly small degrees.

The "front shoulder," for example, is the portion of the deltoid muscle that . . . well, it's on the front. (Give the bodybuilders props for keeping it simple.) That part of the muscle is involved in all forms of bench presses—less on the decline press, somewhat more on the incline press—as well as in dips. It's also heavily involved in shoulder presses. And some bodybuilders do all those exercises, plus special dumbbell exercises for that particular portion of the deltoid. All that work, for a sliver of muscle that's only a few inches long and, at most, an inch wide.

There's more to the deltoid: The middle portion gets worked in any exercise in which you raise your arms to the side or over your head, as in shoulder presses and lateral raises. The rear part helps pull your arms backward, which I'll get into in the next chapter. My point is that you can work the front and middle portions perfectly well with a couple of pushing exercises, one vertical (military press) and one horizontal (bench press). And you'll take care of the rear shoulders with standard pulling exercises.

The other visible and important pushing muscle is the triceps. It's a three-headed muscle that straightens your elbow when it's bent. One part of it—the long head—crosses the shoulder joint, and thus it helps out on some pulling exercises. But don't lose any sleep over that bit of muscle trivia. Your triceps will grow perfectly well without any fancy delineation of function, doing one exercise for the long head, another for the medial head (a flat, thick portion down by your elbow), and still another for the lateral head (the part on the outside of your upper arm that forms the horseshoe shape with the long head). Dips and bench presses work all three heads.

Powerlifters usually do some dedicated exercises that isolate and strengthen their triceps, using heavy barbells and dumbbells. And, given how important triceps are to bench-press performance, you can't blame them. But for the rest of us, it's hard to imagine a few sets of triceps-isolating exercises done on cable machines or with light dumbbells truly adding much size to the arms of someone who's already doing two or three pushing exercises.

FUNCTIONAL IMPORTANCE

Pushing exercises train your body to . . . wait for it . . . push things. And lift things overhead. And throw things. And maybe punch out the occasional obnoxious drunk. (Although you'll still need to incorporate lunging and twisting movements to make the lesson stick.)

TECHNIQUE

On a bench press of any sort, the action is simple: You hold the weight with straight arms above your chest at the start, lower it to your chest, then push straight up to the starting position.

You'll still find some disagreement on a few particulars. Powerlifters, for example, believe that the barbell should come down to the lower chest, which allows the upper arms to get as close as possible to the torso. That creates a stronger platform from which to push the weight off your chest. Serious powerlifters also strive for a higher platform; that's why they employ a nearly parabolic back arch. The goal is to lift the lower chest as high as possible off the bench, thus shortening the distance the bar has to travel to complete a lift.

But even powerlifters disagree about the path the bar should travel. Some recommend a "J lift," in which the bar comes off the chest and up toward the head, then straight up from there. But others, primarily Louie Simmons and the Westside Barbell lifters, believe the bar should go straight up off the lower chest to lockout.

The Westside guys say the shorter the distance the bar has to travel, the better, and that a J lift increases that distance. Other lifters note that the J allows the bar to keep moving, even if part of the movement is horizontal instead of vertical, which can help get the bar through a "sticking point," the place where hopes of a personal-record lift die.

I'll let them fight it out. I think most of us use a combination—straight-up lifts on incline bench presses and shoulder presses, mildly J-shaped lifts on our heaviest barbell flat-bench presses. My advice: Do what your shoulders want to do. You probably won't notice a J-shape on heavy bench presses anyway; your focus is on completing the lift any way possible, and your body will decide if it needs to "J," or if a simple "I" will suffice.

There is some mild controversy about whether to lower a barbell all the way to your chest on the bench press, or even below that if you're using dumbbells. The idea that the full-range-of-motion bench press means death to healthy shoulders used to have near-fanatical believers a few years back. (Their peak was probably the mid-1990s.) It was part of a quasi-religious ideology that weight lifting was inherently dangerous and that the only way to do it safely was to limit the range of motion of most exercises.

But today, I think, the opposite belief is taking hold. As Alwyn has explained it to me, real life forces your joints to go through their full ranges of motion. And it's at those extremes that injuries live. If you go into the gym and teach your body to be strong at select angles, then you aren't doing anything to help your body protect itself at those extreme places. That doesn't mean you have to *extend* your range of motion on the exercises in this book. But we think it's unnecessary, at best, to shorten them beyond what we show here. At worst, it's foolish.

There are caveats, of course; if you're injured and your physical therapist or doctor prescribes a short range of motion near the injury, listen to him or her. Some serious powerlifters use partial ranges of motion with heavier weights than they could

Counterfeit Body Parts

Successful bodybuilders have muscles on top of muscles, lumps and grooves and striations in places where most of us don't even have places. But even with all that going for them, they like to believe they have muscles that don't exist.

One of these is the "inner chest." The idea is that, because it looks cool when pectoral muscles rise like stuffed pitas off the breastbone, there must be special exercises to make this happen.

There aren't. The most cursory glance at an anatomical chart shows that the fibers of the pectoral muscles extend horizontally from the sternum. Thus, the angle of pull can only go one way. Bodybuilders understand this when they do exercises like dumbbell flies, in which they raise and lower weights along the exact line of the muscle fibers. But somehow, many of them believe that it's possible to activate parts of those fibers along a completely different line.

Part of the confusion comes from the fact that the pectoral muscles feel more strained around the sternum on exercises like the dip. That's because they *are* more strained, especially if your muscles are tight and you aren't used to doing dips. But the strain isn't a sign that parts of the fibers are working harder than others and thus will create more growth in that specific spot. You feel a tug because those fibers aren't used to the range of motion and are on the verge of tearing away from the breastbone.

Which won't help your inner chest at all.

use through the full range. That prepares their nervous systems for the shock of using heavier weights. And, of course, bodybuilders do all kinds of exercises in limited ranges of motion, sometimes intentionally. I'm sure they have their reasons . . . other than "too much time on their hands," I mean.

THE EXERCISES

✳ Push-up

USED IN: Break-In

SETUP: Get on the floor, facedown. Support your weight on your toes and hands, with your feet together and your palms flat on the floor and about shoulder-width apart. Your body should form a straight line from neck to ankles. Start with straight arms.

LOWERING: Lower your chest to within an inch or two of the floor, keeping your body in the same alignment.

LIFTING: Push yourself straight up to the starting position.

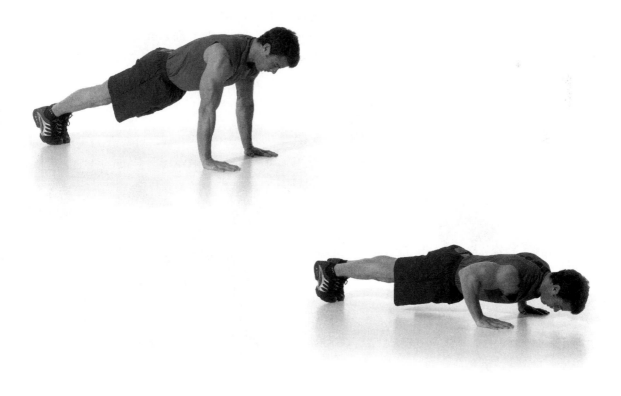

Variations

✳ Explosive push-up *(not shown)*

USED IN: Fat-Loss III

SAME AS ABOVE, EXCEPT . . . Push up so hard that your hands come off the floor. Don't try to do anything fancy, like clap your hands in midair. Just push hard enough to catch the air. If you aren't working out on a carpeted floor with good padding beneath, use a mat to save your hands and wrists.

VERY COOL VARIATION ON THE VARIATION: Push up so hard that your hands and feet come off the floor.

✳ T-push-up

See Chapter 14.

✳ Barbell bench press

USED IN: Hypertrophy II; Strength I, II, and III

SETUP: Set a barbell on the uprights of a bench designed for chest presses. If the uprights are adjustable, make sure they're set high if you have long arms, or low if you

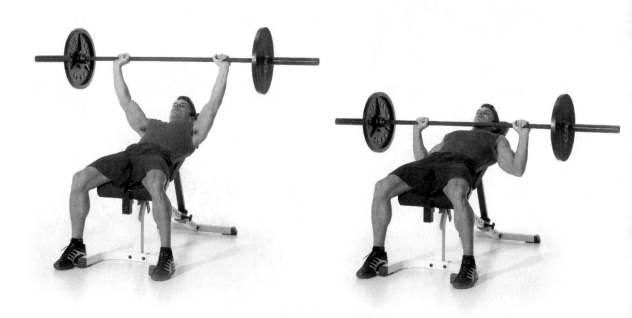

have short arms. Lie on your back on the bench with your feet spread wide and flat on the floor. Grab the bar overhand with a "medium" grip—your hands just outside shoulder-width apart. If you're using an Olympic barbell, you should have your pinkies on the smooth rings cut into the knurled part of the bar. Lift it off the racks (or have a spotter lift it off) and hold it over your chest with your arms straight, including your wrists (don't allow your wrists to bend backward, in other words). Your back should be in its natural arch; if you're an advanced lifter, you can (and should) exaggerate this arch to bring your chest closer to the bar. (As explained in Chapter 8, we shot this on a bench without uprights to make it easier to see the exercise performed. We also used an incline bench for the main photographs here for further clarity.)

LOWERING: Lower the bar to your sternum, just below the bottom of your pectoral muscles.

LIFTING: Push straight up. Make sure you bring the bar down to the same point on your sternum each time.

Variations

✳ Barbell incline bench press *(shown in photos on page 139)*

USED IN: Hypertrophy III

SAME AS ABOVE, EXCEPT . . . Set the bench at an incline between 15 and 30 degrees. Lower the bar to your middle chest instead of the base of your sternum. The higher the angle, the higher on your chest you'll bring the bar.

✳ Barbell close-grip bench press *(not shown)*

USED IN: Hypertrophy I

SAME AS ABOVE, EXCEPT . . . You'll start with your hands closer together; you want your thumbs about twelve inches apart.

VERY COOL VARIATION ON THE VARIATIONS: Try incline close-grip bench presses.

✳ Dumbbell bench press

USED IN: Fat-Loss III; Strength I

SETUP: Grab a pair of dumbbells and lie on a flat bench, with your body and feet positioned as they are in the barbell bench press (see page 136). Hold the dumbbells straight over your chest, with your palms turned toward your feet.

LOWERING: Lower the weights to your chest. The edges of the dumbbells should just graze the outside-middle parts of your pectorals. (Everyone will use slightly different angles and ranges of motion on this exercise; in the end, it's all the same exercise.)

LIFTING: Push the weights straight up to the starting position.

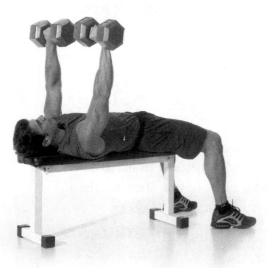

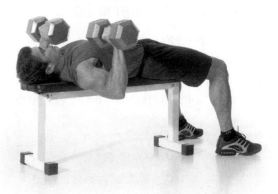

<u>Variation</u>

✳ Dumbbell incline bench press

USED IN: Fat-Loss I; Hypertrophy I; Hypertrophy II (palms facing each other); Strength II (normal grip)

SAME AS ABOVE, EXCEPT . . . Set the bench on an incline of about 30 to 45 degrees. (The angle is steeper than it was on the barbell bench press because dumbbells are easier on your shoulders.) In Hypertrophy II, you'll turn your palms in toward each other. That'll bring your elbows in closer to your torso, which should activate your triceps and front deltoids a bit more and your chest a bit less.

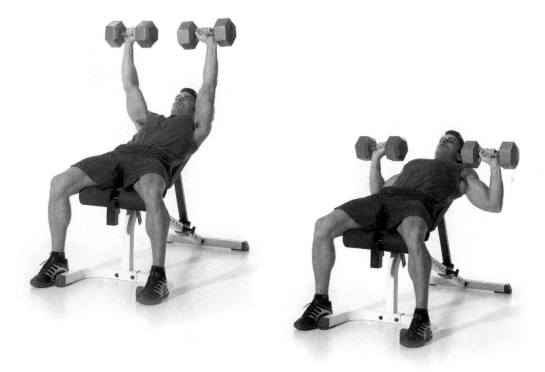

✳ Barbell shoulder press

USED IN: Hypertrophy II; Strength I and III

SET-UP: If you can, set up a barbell in a squat rack so you can lift it off supports at about shoulder level. (If you can't, you'll have to "clean" the bar from the floor, described below.) Grab the bar overhand, with your hands just beyond shoulder-width apart. (Feel free to adjust your grip width for shoulder-joint comfort.) Stand, holding the bar in front of and just above your shoulders. You want your body in an athletic posture: feet shoulder-width apart, knees slightly bent, torso tight with a natural arch in your lower back, eyes looking straight ahead.

LIFTING: Push the weight straight up, moving your head back until the bar rises past it. At the top you want straight arms and the bar directly above your ears.

LOWERING: Slowly lower the bar along the same path to the starting position.

IF YOU HAVE TO CLEAN THE WEIGHT FROM THE FLOOR: Set up as you would for a high pull (see Chapter 14). The movement is the same, except at the end you flip your elbows under the bar so the bar ends up on your front shoulders. Now set your torso for the press, as described.

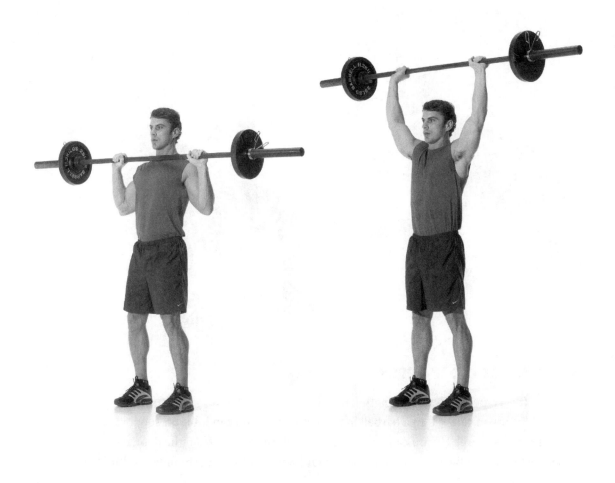

Variation

✳ Barbell push press

USED IN: Fat-Loss II; Hypertrophy III; Strength II and III

SAME AS ABOVE, EXCEPT . . . You're going to use momentum to get the bar moving off your shoulders. Bend your knees and hips, as if you were going to jump. Then . . . jump, pushing the bar upward as your knees and hips straighten. You can come all the way up on your toes.

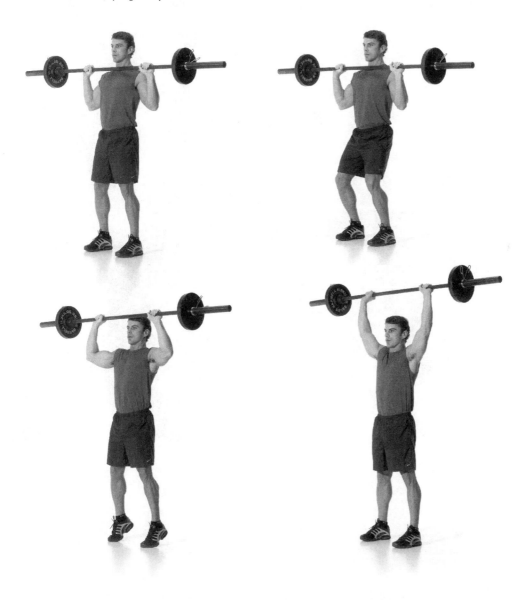

✳ Dumbbell shoulder press

USED IN: Fat-Loss III; Hypertrophy I; Strength I and II

SETUP: Grab a pair of dumbbells and hold them at the edges of your shoulders, palms facing out. Posture is athletic, as described for the barbell shoulder press.

LIFTING: Push the weights straight up over your shoulders (not up and toward each other so they clank; the movement takes tension off the shoulders and triceps, and the noise is obnoxious).

LOWERING: Lower them along the same path to the edges of your shoulders.

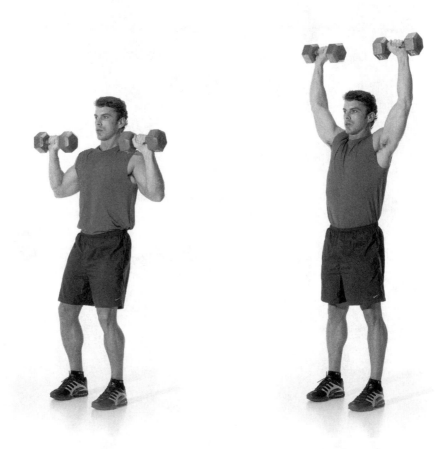

<u>Variations</u>

✳ Dumbbell one-arm shoulder press *(not shown)*

USED IN: Break-In

SAME AS ABOVE, EXCEPT . . . Start with your palms facing each other, and lift with one arm at a time.

VERY COOL VARIATION ON THE VARIATION: Bend to the sides as you lift—to the left as you lift with your right arm, to the right as you lift with your left. That adds some work for your torso.

✳ Dumbbell push press *(not shown)*

USED IN: Fat-Loss I and III

SAME AS ABOVE, EXCEPT . . . As with the barbell push press, you dip your knees, and use momentum to push the weights up.

✳ Dumbbell Chek press *(not shown)*

USED IN: Hypertrophy II

SAME AS ABOVE, EXCEPT . . . Stand holding the dumbbells in front of your torso with your palms facing each other. Your upper arms are perpendicular to your torso and parallel to the floor, with your elbows bent 90 degrees. Press straight up from there. At the top, swing your elbows out to the sides so your palms are facing forward. Lower the weights to your shoulders, then swing your elbows back so they're out in front of your torso again.

✳ Dip

USED IN: Hypertrophy II and III

SETUP: Find a station for parallel-bar dips. (It's often part of another apparatus. At my gym, for example, the handles are part of the captain's chair, an ab-training device.) Grab the bars overhand, meaning your knuckles are facing out. You want to start with your body elevated and your arms straight. If the apparatus doesn't have a step that makes it easier to get into this position, you may have to jump from the floor to get your arms straight. You want your torso leaning forward slightly. Bend your knees and cross your feet behind you.

LOWERING: How far you lower yourself depends on your level of experience, strength, and shoulder-joint integrity. Some guys can go all the way down until biceps meet forearms. Others can barely bend their elbows 90 degrees. We don't recommend going lower than the point at which your upper arms are parallel to the floor.

LIFTING: Push back up to the starting position.

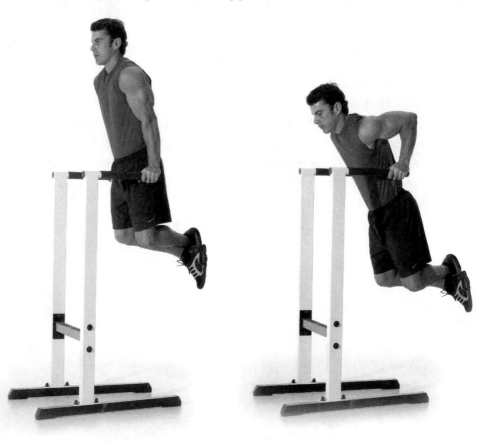

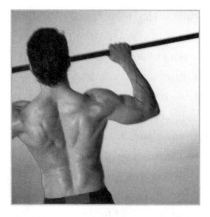

Pull

W̲HEN I WAS GROWING UP, about a million years ago, we would describe certain guys as having "forearms like a milkman." It was not only a compliment (believe me, I can think of a few ways to spin that phrase the other direction) toward men with large, muscular arms, it was a description of a way of life that, like the profession of delivering bottles of milk to people's homes, has mostly disappeared.

People used to do some amount of physical work to earn their paychecks. You could see it in their appearances. Yes, there were fat men back then (my father was among the fattest), but there weren't many with what we now describe as a "schlumpy" posture: shoulders rounded forward, bellies pushed out.

In fact, if you saw a guy with a protruding belly, chances are he pulled his shoulders back to compensate. Nowadays, a guy with schlumpy shoulders will do the opposite: He'll roll the top of his pelvis backward, and the bottom of his pelvis forward, which flattens his lower back and makes it easier to sit for extended amounts of time with those shoulders hunched forward.

And sitting, of course, is the modern condition. We sit to drive, to peck on our computers, to eat. Hell, go into any gym, and count how many people sit throughout their entire workouts. They start on a recumbent bike, and then "do the machines" (in flagrant violation of New Rule #7), virtually all of which *require* sitting (seated lat pulldown, seated horizontal chest press, seated machine crunch, seated row . . .). Among the few exercises that allow standing is the cable triceps extension. And even that has evolved in the past decade or so from an exercise in which you generally stand facing the weight stack to one in which you rest your back against a pad, facing out away from the weight stack. That's about as close to sitting as you can get without actually sitting.

If you had to pick one of the six basic movements as more crucial than the others in fighting the continued disintegration of adult posture, you'd be wise to choose the pull. Driving and typing involve a forward reach—sort of a permanently enabled pushing motion—but modern life has no corresponding movements to compensate.

Generations ago, physical labor involved pulling. There were the milkmen, of course, but also the pre-automation factory workers and farmers. Many jobs—perhaps most—required that someone be able to grab a box or barrel or stack of something, pull it closer to his torso, and then transport it somewhere else. If the object was on the floor, the worker had to perform a movement very much like the bent-over row we do in gyms today. (Followed, of course, by a deadlift-type movement to stand upright.)

Then there were the jobs that involved climbing up ladders, using a combination of pulling and lunging movements. Today, aside from some construction positions, few of us have to climb ladders.

Now, the last thing I'd ever do is claim that the exercises in this section will fix postural problems created by eight or ten or twelve hours a day of sitting. They won't. In fact, a study published in the *Journal of Strength and Conditioning Research* in 2001 threw cold water all over the idea that targeted exercises can reverse bad posture. If you're sitting for ten hours a day and doing posture-perfecting exercises for ten minutes, of course your body is going to respond to the former more than the latter. What they can do is give you awareness of the way the muscles in your upper back are supposed to feel when they're pulling your shoulders back. From there, it's up to you to remind yourself to square your shoulders.

But at least the exercises are a start.

THE MUSCLES

The most important pulling muscles act on three joints:

- Your latissimus dorsi ("lats") and rear deltoids act on your shoulder joints, pulling your arms back and/or down when they're extended overhead or in front of you.
- Your trapezius has three distinct functions, all of which involve moving your shoulder blades. Your upper trapezius moves them up (as in a shrug), your middle traps move them closer together (as in a row), and your lower traps pull them down (which happens in a pull-up or lat pulldown).
- Your biceps and other assorted muscles in your upper and lower arms bend your elbows.

Of all these, the contraction of your middle traps—called "scapular retraction"—has the most effect on your posture. A model I worked with at *Men's Health* offered the best description of it I've ever come across: He said guys should walk like they're Superman, with their capes flowing behind them. To do that, you not only have to pull your shoulders together in back, you have to pull them down, too; Superman would never walk around with hunched shoulders. The Superman strut instantly makes you feel taller, stronger, and more in control of your environment.

Alwyn's *New Rules* workouts have plenty of exercises in which you'll be instructed to perform scapular retraction. But one exercise you won't see in his workouts is the one-arm dumbbell row. If you've spent any time at all around dumbbells—and I mean both kinds—you'll have seen this exercise performed countless times.

Typically, it looks like this: The exerciser rests his left knee and hand on a bench, and then rows a dumbbell with his right hand up to his right side. If it's an older woman doing the exercise, the dumbbell is usually the weight of a Kleenex box, but the woman still does the row slowly and deliberately, as if one false move with that paperweight will cause her entire skeleton to crumble. If it's a bodybuilder doing it, the dumbbell weighs more than Catholic guilt, and he's using almost every muscle in his body to move it six inches or so.

What neither type of lifter, or anyone in between, is likely to do is perform a scapular retraction. The old, frail woman has almost no tension on her muscles; the weight is so light that she can perform a facsimile of the exercise using nothing but her arm and rear-shoulder muscles. The bodybuilder is using middle- and lower-body muscles to generate momentum to get all that iron moving. That involves a torso twist, which prevents his trapezius from getting involved. His shoulder blades don't need to get any closer to each other, since he's using his core and gluteal muscles to rotate his shoulders upward.

Alwyn chose a cool variation on that exercise to get around the problem. In the two-point dumbbell row, you'll stand on both feet, bend over at the hips, hold a dumbbell with one hand, and keep the other arm behind your back. From that position, you have to focus on stabilizing your torso, instead of feeling free to twist it. You should feel it in all your back muscles, from top to bottom.

Get good at it—along with the other rowing variations Alwyn includes in the *New Rules* programs—and you won't have any trouble feeling the flow from Superman's cape.

FUNCTIONAL IMPORTANCE

As I said at the start of this chapter, part of the problem with modern life is that there's very little pulling involved, unless you do a lot of physical labor in your free time—construction, yard work, recreational steer-roping (relaxes me!).

In sports, climbing and rowing involve pulls, as does wrestling. Sailing involves all sorts of pulls; nautically minded friends assure me that, on the most windy days, sports like windsurfing challenge your back and arm muscles about as much as they can be challenged. Dragging a kayak or wind sail into shore is yet another pulling challenge.

Perhaps the biggest benefit of doing pulling exercises in the gym, aside from improved postural awareness, is that you teach your body how to do it without getting hurt. A study by Stuart McGill** showed that veteran firefighters were able to push and pull loads with hardly any stress on their lower backs.

The other group used in the study—college students with no particular experience or training in the movements tested—experienced all kinds of back strain. But the firemen knew how to use their entire bodies in movement sequences that kept their backs safe.

And that's exactly what Alwyn and I hope you get out of the exercises in this book, and especially those in this chapter.

TECHNIQUE

Alwyn's workouts feature two types of pulling exercises (well, three, actually, but the high pull takes a bit of explanation; you'll find it with the combo-movement exercises in Chapter 14). For simplicity's sake, let's use Ian King's terminology and call them "vertical" and "horizontal" pulling.

Both types of pulls start with a scapular movement.

The key to the vertical pull—a category that includes lat pulldowns, chin-ups, and pull-ups—is an initial downward movement of your scapulae. In English, that means you start by pulling your shoulder blades down and together.

Then you engage your lats and rear deltoids, which pull your upper arms down and back slightly. Your biceps and forearm muscles kick in last, bending your elbows so you can get your chin over the bar, or the pulldown bar to your chest. You don't have to pay attention to the sequence, of course; it happens on its own.

A similar sequence occurs with the horizontal pulls, which include bent-over and seated rows. This time, the first movement is scapular retraction, your shoulder blades coming together in the middle of your back. (You can always tell when someone is nearing the end of a set of cable seated rows. His shoulders start to rise up, a sign that his middle traps are officially fried.) Then the lats and rear delts engage to pull your arms back, and then your arms kick in.

On both types of pulls, you want to keep your hips and lower back tight and engaged but not put them in motion. Thus, no leaning back on the lat pulldown or cable seated row.

A real danger with the seated rows comes when you allow your torso to lean forward and your lower back to slip out of its natural arch. You're begging for a spinal-disc injury when you do that.

Pull-up or Pulldown?

This rule is simple: If you can do pull-ups or chin-ups for the designated number of repetitions, choose them. If you can't (and few of us can, when the workout calls for more than ten reps), do a lat pulldown with a comparable grip—underhand for chin-ups, overhand for pull-ups, mixed-grip when that's called for. Chin-ups and pull-ups are total-body exercises, since you have to contract everything to keep your body balanced when you're hanging from the bar. Pulldowns work the upper body perfectly well but allow the lower body to take a break.

THE EXERCISES

✳ Lat pulldown

USED IN: All programs (see "Pull-up or Pulldown?" on page 149 for an explanation)

SETUP: Attach the appropriate bar to the high pulley of the lat-pulldown station. Grab the bar with the designated grip (if the workout chart doesn't specify, use an overhand grip that's just outside shoulder width). Position yourself with your knees under the pads, if the apparatus you're using has them. Start with your arms straight,

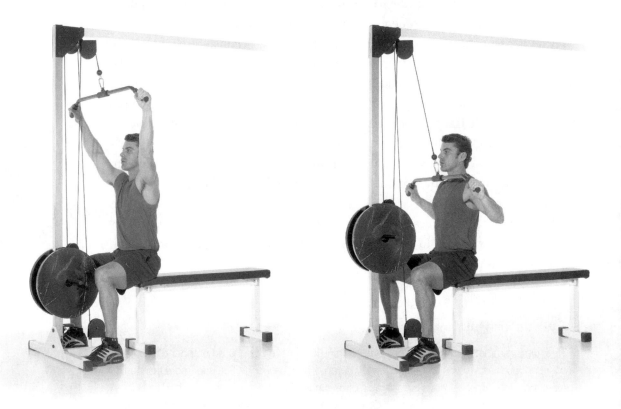

Win One for the Gripper

Every well-equipped gym offers a variety of attachments for rows and lat pulldowns. These handles allow every possible type of grip—overhand, underhand, and whatever lies in between. Let's look at how those various grips affect your muscles.

Your forearm has two bones, the radius and the ulna. The two of them are parallel to each other when you take a palms-up grip, with the ulna on the inside (above the pinkie) and the radius on the thumb-side. That alignment puts your biceps in their strongest position.

When you rotate your hands inward so your palms face each other, you have what's called a "neutral" or, if you want to get *really* geeky, "semi-supinated" grip. Your forearms are in a very strong position with this grip, since you've now fully engaged two muscles: the brachialis, a thick, strong muscle that lies between the biceps and your upper-arm bone, and the brachioradialis, your biggest forearm muscle. The biceps are in a weakened position here, but they still contribute.

If you rotate your palms all the way around so you have an overhand grip, you've twisted your radius all the way around your ulna, so the radius is now on the inside. That puts your biceps in the weakest position of all, although the brachialis and brachioradialis are still strong in this position.

Many believe that a wider grip on pullups and pulldowns builds a wider back. It's not really true, since the main upper-back muscles—the lats and traps—don't engage differently with different arm widths. They pull your arms down and shoulder blades together in all these exercises.

But a wider grip does force your arms out farther from your torso, which challenges your rear deltoids more. And the wide, overhand grip does put your arm muscles in a relatively weak position, meaning the lats might have to work harder, even if the range of motion is shorter with a wider grip.

torso upright. (It's okay to lean back a few degrees at the start, as long as you can hold that position throughout the movement.)

LIFTING: Initiate the pull by squeezing your shoulder blades together in back. Pull the bar to your upper chest without leaning back to generate momentum. It's helpful to envision pushing your chest up toward the bar; that puts your upper-back muscles in their strongest position.

LOWERING: Return the bar to the starting position, keeping it under control.

Variations

These are easy to figure out from the workout charts:

- "Wide-grip" means you use the widest possible grip on the longest bar. (The grips on these bars are angled downward slightly.)
- "Close-grip" means the triangle-shaped attachment; your palms will face each other with your hands just a few inches apart.
- "Underhand-grip" means you grab any bar with your palms up and your hands shoulder-width apart.
- "Mixed-grip" means a combination overhand-underhand grip on the bar. Alternate on each set, so if you start with your right hand over the bar on the first set, it'll be under the bar on the next. If you're doing an uneven number of sets, change grips halfway through the final set so you get equal work for both sides of your body.

The Truth About Arm Curls

Show this program to any serious bodybuilder, and he'll scoff at the lack of arm exercises. Nothing is more sacred to the bodybuilding mythos than the idea that small muscles designed to assist bigger muscles in multi-joint movements need their own special exercises, if not entire workouts.

I confess: Even I was convinced that those arm exercises must do something. My position was that they represented a lot of time and effort for a pretty small reward.

But when I went through some studies recently, I was surprised to find that this is only true for beginners. Advanced lifters don't necessarily get any increase in arm size from arm-isolating exercises.

Let's start with a 1993 study published in the *Journal of Applied Physiology.* The researchers put elderly men through twelve weeks of heavy-duty training. They did two biceps workouts a week, consisting of four exercises: three sets each of barbell, dumbbell, and hammer curls (a hammer curl is a dumbbell curl in which you keep your palms turned toward each other instead of pointing up toward the ceiling), plus four sets of curls on a Cybex machine.

The oldies quickly became goodies: The volume of their biceps increased 14 percent, while their biceps "peak" ("the point of maximal girth of the muscle") swelled a whopping 23 percent.

If I thought I could get those results from twenty-six sets of curls a week, I'd be right in there curling away with the meatheads and mooks. But I almost certainly can't. That's because, when studies look specifically at changes in arm girth in *experienced* lifters, they don't find any.

Let's start with the same team that performed the aforementioned study. The year before, in the same journal, the researchers showed that competitive bodybuilders saw no increase in arm girth after a twenty-four-week training program.

Their conclusion: "These data suggest that the extent of any change in muscle mass or muscle fiber characteristics is minimal after a bodybuilder of either gender has attained a high degree of muscle mass and a highly competitive status."

Here's another, more recent study, published in 2002 in the *Journal of Strength and Conditioning Research*. The object of the study was to look at a specific training technique, which isn't worth describing here. However, only half the experienced lifters in the study were using that technique. The rest were doing their exercises the conventional way. And neither group saw any changes in arm size in nine weeks.

Of course, a good trainer can always find some way to increase a dedicated lifter's muscle size—he'll find some kind of unique stimulus the lifter hasn't tried before. But chances are about 100 percent that any increase in arm size in a seasoned ironhead would be accompanied by increases in the size of all the muscles surrounding the shoulder joint—delts, pecs, lats, traps. Even then, the changes in size wouldn't be dramatic, unless the lifter had been starving himself before the program began (thus deliberately shrinking his muscles so that they would grow faster when he started eating again) or unless he had overeaten to the point that he had gained a lot of fat along with the muscle size.

Bottom line: Curls are mostly for newbies and juicers. Unless you have a specific reason for doing arm-isolating exercises, save your time and energy for other pursuits.

✳ Pull-up and chin-up

USED IN: All programs (see "Pull-up or Pull-down?" on page 149)

SETUP: Grab the chin-up bar with the appropriate grip:

- overhand and just outside shoulder-width for pull-ups
- underhand and at shoulder-width, or a bit inside that, for chin-ups (shown on this page)
- overhand and well outside shoulder-width for "wide-grip"
- well inside shoulder-width for "close-grip" (underhand for chin-ups, overhand for pull-ups)
- one hand over and one hand under the bar for "mixed grip."

Hang from the bar at arm's length, with your lower legs crossed behind you.

LIFTING: Pull yourself up to the bar. Your chin should go over for chin-ups; for pull-ups, go as high as you can.

LOWERING: Lower your body along the same path.

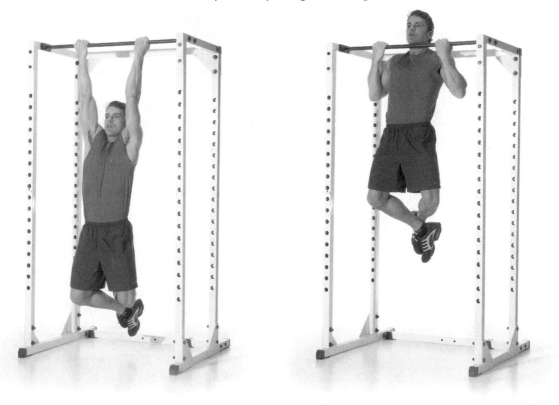

✳ Cable seated row

USED IN: Fat-Loss I, II, and III; Hypertrophy I and II; Strength I, II, and III

SETUP: Attach the appropriate bar to the low cable of the rowing station. Grab it with the appropriate grip (if the workout chart doesn't specify, use an overhand grip that's just outside shoulder width). Set your feet against the supports, if your gym's apparatus has them. You want your knees bent slightly and your torso perpendicular to the floor, with your lower back in its natural arch and your eyes focused straight ahead. Start with your arms straight and shoulders down (not hunched).

LIFTING: Initiate the pull by squeezing your shoulder blades together in back. Pull the bar to your abdomen (unless the workout chart specifies "to chest"; see below).

LOWERING: Return the bar to the starting position, keeping it under control.

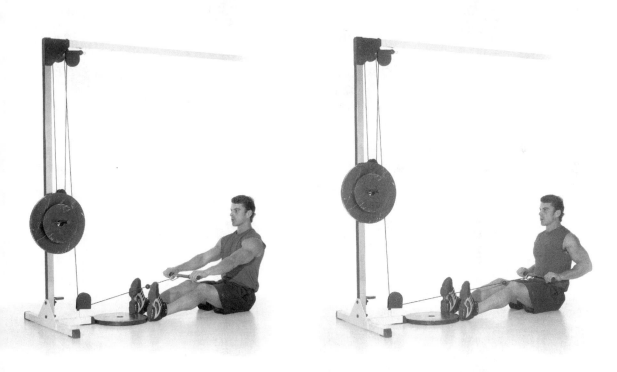

Variations

Again, the variations are clear from the charts:

- "Wide-grip" means you use the longest possible bar, which you'll usually have to commandeer from the lat-pulldown station.

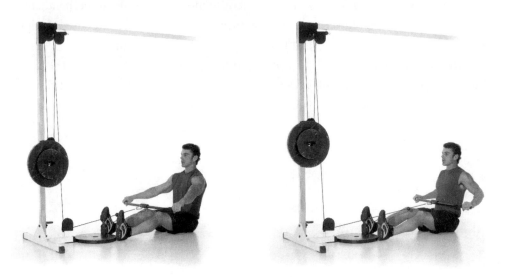

- To "chest" means you pull the designated bar up higher, which adds more challenge for your traps and rear shoulders.

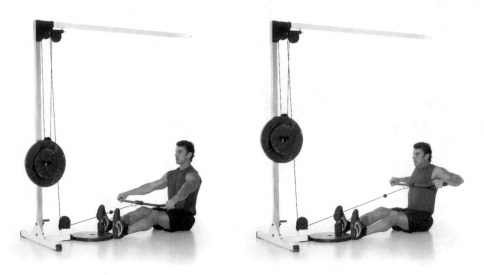

✳ Two-point dumbbell row

USED IN: Fat-Loss III

SETUP: Grab a dumbbell in your left hand (or your right hand if you're left-handed). Stand with your feet shoulder-width apart, knees slightly bent, and your non-working hand behind your back. Bend forward at the hips as far as you can while keeping the natural arch in your lower back. Hold the dumbbell in a neutral grip (if you were standing up straight with your arm at your side, your palm would face your thigh), with your arm straight down from your left shoulder.

LIFTING: Pull the dumbbell up to your side, with your elbow finishing above and behind your torso.

LOWERING: Lower the weight along the same path. Finish all your reps, then switch arms and repeat.

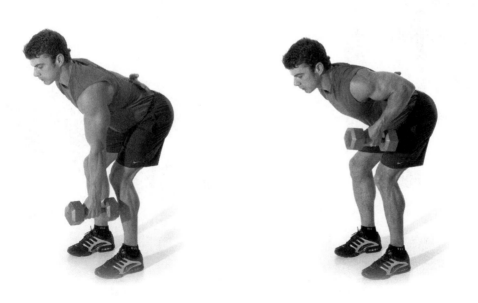

✳ Two-point dumbbell row with elbow out

USED IN: Break-In

SAME AS ABOVE, EXCEPT . . . You'll start with your palm facing behind you. Pull up and out to your side, so your upper arm is nearly perpendicular to your torso at the top of the movement. This will make the exercise more of a challenge to your traps and rear shoulders.

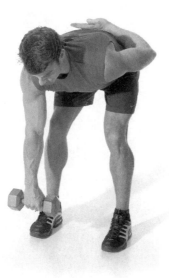

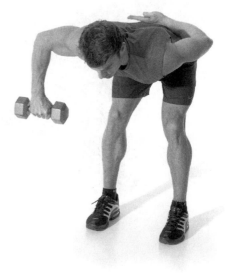

✳ Barbell bent-over row

USED IN: Hypertrophy III; Strength I, II, and III

SETUP: Grab a barbell with an overhand grip that's just outside shoulder width. Stand with your feet shoulder width apart, knees slightly bent. Bend at the hips as far as you can without losing the natural arch in your lower back. The bar should hang straight down from your shoulders.

LIFTING: Pull the bar up to your abdomen.

LOWERING: Slowly lower it along the same path.

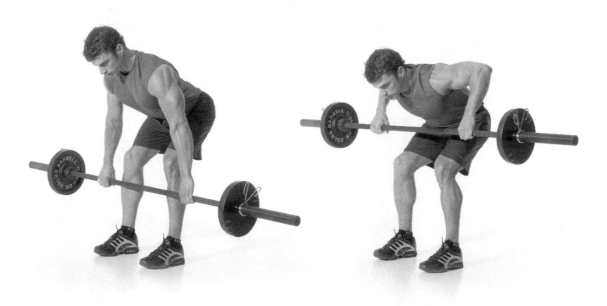

Variation

✳ Barbell reverse-grip bent-over row *(not shown)*

USED IN: Hypertrophy II

SAME AS ABOVE, EXCEPT . . . Grab the bar with an underhand, shoulder-width grip. This puts more emphasis on your biceps (a horrible sacrifice, we know).

✳ Towel biceps curl

USED IN: Hypertrophy II

SETUP: You'll need to bring two hand towels with you to the gym, if your gym doesn't have them. Grab two dumbbells, and stand them on end so they're vertical instead of horizontal. Wrap a towel around the inside top edge of one, and grab the ends of the towel in one hand. The dumbbell should be cradled securely in the middle of the towel. Do the same with the other dumbbell, and grab the towel ends with your other hand. Now stand with your arms at your sides, holding the ends of the two towels with the dumbbells hanging below.

LIFTING: Keeping your back in its natural position and your entire torso tight (to prevent any movement that'll generate momentum and make the lift easier), pull the weights up as high as you can without moving your upper arms forward.

LOWERING: Slowly lower the weights along the same path.

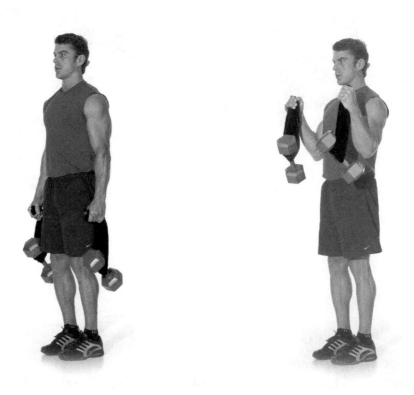

✳ **Dumbbell clean** (*not shown*)

USED IN: Hypertrophy III

SET-UP: Grab a pair of dumbbells and stand holding them at your sides, your palms facing in. You want your body set in an athletic posture, with feet shoulder-width apart and knees slightly bent.

LIFTING: Dip your knees and hips, as if you were going to jump, then reverse direction, straightening your knees and hips as you come up on your toes and shrug your shoulders. As the weights are moving upward, pull them up with your arms and shoulders so the ends of the dumbbells land on top of your shoulders. It's okay to bend your knees and hips again to dip under the weights and "catch" them. Stand straight again to finish the lift.

LOWERING: Lower the weights to the starting position and set your body for the next rep. Focus on perfect form for each repetition, generating maximum power, rather than trying to get into rhythmic repetitions.

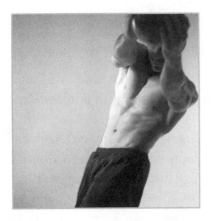

13

Twist

This chapter is the trickiest of all, since it's going to include almost everything that you would describe as "ab" training. And yet, very little abdominal training—in this book or elsewhere—requires actual twisting.

So my logic here mandates a few hops, steps, and jumps, and by the time I'm finished I'll be out of breath and you still may not agree with my thesis. I'll accept that risk.

Here's the central problem for me: Traditional abdominal exercises, those based on crunches and sit-ups, don't involve an essential human movement. In fact, for lack of a better phrase, they represent the *absence* of essential human movement. And yet, we all do them, and some of them are included in this program.

When we talk about crunches, what we're really talking about is a forward bend, the opposite of the deadlift movement. But in sports and real life, a forward bend isn't performed against gravity. There's never a moment in which that movement, in isolation, is necessarily to transport your body, to transport an object, to attack an enemy, or to fend off an attack. You don't need it to build shelter or tear down someone else's shelter. It won't help you kill an animal or escape from one.

And yet the ability to brace your abdominals is crucial to performing all six of the human movements safely and effectively:

Squat and deadlift: This is simple: If your middle body isn't braced, if those muscles surrounding your spine aren't in a high state of tension, your back loses its shape and something ruptures. You're screwed.

Lunge and twist: If you can't hold your torso in place, or move it in a controlled twisting motion while your legs are splayed apart, you'll be unable to maintain your balance, and you'll fall or tear something. And you're screwed.

Push and pull: You can't execute either of these movements without a stable platform. Your feet form a base for your legs, which are the pillars that hold up the platform. But your middle body—hips, pelvis, spine—*is* the platform. If that platform is moving randomly, you can't execute a pull without risk of hurting yourself. You can't execute a push at all. And, of course, you're screwed.

Further complicating all this:

The middle body isn't merely a platform, like a slab of concrete that can be made more or less stable. It's the nerve center, the part that allows communication between the parts that need a platform—the arms and the shoulder complex—and the parts that support the platform.

So, with that established (or the issue thoroughly confused; I'll let you decide), let's talk about the twist itself.

In the gym, we tend to think of twisting motions as specific exercises. There are the more sophisticated ones, like the Russian twist and its variations that Alwyn has included in these programs. Then there are the really, really stupid things like the old "twist with a broomstick" exercise that dumbbots used to do back in the age of butt-floss and leg warmers. The broomstick twist did one of two things: You either wasted your time by doing an exercise in which your muscles were unchallenged by either gravity or any kind of external resistance, or you applied external resistance—I can remember seeing guys twist with loaded barbells—and did one of the most danger-ous things you could possibly do to your spine.

Then there are the real-life and sports uses of twisting motions. If you sat down in the morning and recorded all the times you twisted at the hips, waist, or shoulders throughout a day, you wouldn't get much else done. You'd start with whatever twist it took to reach into your desk drawer and pull out a pad and pencil. And once you started, like I said, it would be hard to know when to stop. Every time the phone rings, every time you reach for a pencil or Post-it, every time you turn to check out the new intern walking past . . .

In sports, the twists are more dramatic. In basketball, you could drive the lane and end up with your legs going one direction while your upper body twists in the opposite direction to dish off to a teammate. In football, you could jump to catch a pass, only to see the ball get tipped, forcing you to reach back behind you to attempt a reception. And all this could happen while you're bracing for a collision with a defensive back.

Your body instinctively knows how to do two or three things at once; you can walk and chew gum at the same time. But that doesn't mean you can do those things at full speed, with your body contorted to the limits of its reach and flexibility, while simultaneously bracing for impact, without a high risk of injury.

That's where conditioning comes in. That's why you work to make sure your abdominal muscles are not just strong in isolation but also strong during various kinds of motion. And that's why we train the midsection two ways: with exercises like crunches and leg raises, the goal of which is to make your middle strong enough to resist movements you don't want; and in twisting-type motions, in which the goal is to train it to execute safely the movements you *do* want.

None of this means that the only result you'll get from these exercises is a functional benefit. You'll be able to see the difference, too. Applying direct resistance to muscles makes them grow. So while Alwyn has lofty, function-friendly reasons for prescribing exercises like Swiss-ball crunches and hanging leg raises, both of us know that those exercises will create bigger, more visible abdominal muscles. If you're lean enough to see them, they'll look cool. If not, they'll still work better than they did before.

THE MUSCLES

The body-partists tend to see midsection muscles—as they see all muscles—as distinct entities, to be trained in isolation. So they talk about "upper" abs (trained with crunches), "lower abs" (worked with reverse crunches and hanging leg raises), "obliques" (trained with side bends and twisting crunches), and "lower back" (trained with back extensions).

Trainers who emphasize function fall prey to some isolationism, too. They just talk about different muscles in isolation.

One of their favorites is the transverse abdominis (TA). Until recently, I, too, thought this strap of muscle, the innermost layer of your abdominal wall, had an important function that required it to be trained with transverse-specific exercises. But then I read Dr. Stuart McGill's *Ultimate Back Fitness and Performance,* and I changed my mind. McGill says that the interest in the TA started with research showing that people with back injuries have problems activating their TA when they most need it. This is true, McGill says, but it's also true that people with back injuries have problems activating *all* muscles in proper sequences and with sufficient force. That's the biggest challenge with back injuries: They set off a chain reaction that uncoordinates muscles seemingly unrelated to the original injury.

McGill is adamant about this: "Task and motion must be trained—not a specific muscle."

Your abdominal wall is really three walls: You have an outer layer (external obliques), middle layer (internal obliques), and inner layer (transverse abdominis). They're anchored at the back by your spine, which itself is supported on either side by

Suck It Up, but Don't Suck 'Em In

Some midsection myths have been debunked over and over. Does anybody, for example, still believe that doing hundreds of crunches a day will somehow, magically, give you a thinner waist?

But one mythic notion still holds some currency: Pulling your abs in toward your belly button provides a sturdier abdominal wall, and thus more protection for your spine.

I call this the "taffy hypothesis." If you press down on a section of a piece of taffy, thus compressing it and making it thinner, is it stronger at the point of compression? No, of course not. You can hold it by the top, by the bottom, or anywhere in between, and the taffy will always be weakest at the place where it's thinnest.

Dr. McGill and others have argued this point for years. In 2004, researchers at the University of Nebraska Medical Center in Omaha demonstrated it in a study published in the *Journal of Orthopaedic and Sports Physical Therapy.* They had exercisers try to do crunches with their abs either sucked in toward their spine, or "braced," as I describe under "Technique," page 167. Those with braced abs actually had stronger contractions in their rectus abdominis muscles. The ones who sucked them in did work their obliques harder, so it's conceivable that the suck-up maneuver could be construed as a decent way to train those muscles.

But the obliques get involved in all abdominal movements whether you want them to or not. If you're going to do a crunch-type exercise at all, you may want to keep your abs braced and use the exercise to build and strengthen the six-pack.

your spinal erectors, a series of muscles that run up your back in parallel columns. On the front, you have your rectus abdominis, the six-pack muscle.

While each has its own duties, the key is that all work together to protect your spine and internal organs.

A better question, I think, is why we have that strong, visible, and unique rectus abdominis in the front of our midsection.

We all know the rectus bends your torso forward. The fibers run vertically, which means it's perfectly designed for that function. But I've already established (or tried my damnedest to establish) that forward bending against gravity or some other kind of resistance isn't a particularly important task—certainly nothing more than a subcategory of the big six movements.

But surely our bodies wouldn't evolve to include a muscle like that, and then give it nothing of consequence to do.

Think back to what I wrote earlier in this chapter, about how your middle body is both a "platform" and a "nerve center." In its role as a platform, it has to be ready for a challenge from any direction—from above, below, or anything in between. It's even designed to absorb forces coming from inside.

Let's say you're doing a squat with a maximum load on your shoulders. For me, that would be about 300 pounds; for you, it could be anything from 50 to 500. Doesn't matter. Your body copes with that load by compressing everything inside your abdomen to help shore up your spine. So while we typically think of the TA and obliques as the belt that shores up this visceral mass, your rectus has to play a part.

In other words, your rectus can take pressure from the inside, as well as from the outside, as it would if you were tightening up to absorb a punch.

The other way your rectus absorbs pressure is from the sides. That is, when you twist with your powerful oblique muscles—and believe me, your obliques are very strong—your rectus abdominis is tasked with keeping your torso together. That, according to McGill, is why it has a beaded shape, broken up by extraordinarily tough bands of connective tissue. Without something there in the middle, your obliques are strong enough to twist your body apart like taffy.

Thus, when you do twisting exercises in your workouts, you're not only training your obliques to get stronger, you're also training your rectus to get stronger at resisting that twist.

Get on the Ball

Some guys just hate Swiss balls. I'm not sure, exactly, what causes the animus. Maybe it's the color of the balls, or the fact women are more likely to use them. But a more likely explanation, I think, is a cultural divide. If you're comfortable with weight rooms the way they are now, with the barbells and dumbbells and benches and machines used just so, the Swiss ball is a foreign intruder, like the annoying person at the office who starts talking about politics on Monday morning when everyone else is analyzing the weekend's football games.

Among experts, there's lots of skepticism about the value of doing *everything* on a Swiss ball, from chest presses to squats. (Yes, some people do get up on the balls and do squats. No, I'm not sure how they do it, either.) But at least one Swiss-ball exercise deserves its inflated reputation.

In a 2000 study in the journal *Physical Therapy,* Spanish researchers compared four types of abdominal crunches. The Swiss-ball crunch, by a long shot, made the abdominal muscles work the hardest. The six-pack muscle, the rectus abdominis, worked twice as hard on the Swiss ball as it did in the traditional floor crunch. Even better, the external obliques got more than four times as much work on the ball.

So even if you stick to standards for every other exercise in the lexicon, the Swiss-ball crunch makes it worth your while to cross over to the other side.

FUNCTIONAL IMPORTANCE

Every human movement involves communication between your upper and lower body, and the midsection is the router that makes sure the communications are received and acted upon.

Still, there are some specific tasks that are highly twist-dependent. In baseball, throwing and hitting both require powerful trunk twists. Same for racquet sports. And a round of golf is twist after twist after twist—the worse you are, the more you twist, which I can report from personal experience.

TECHNIQUE

The wild card in all this is your spine. It's entirely possible to weaken the connective tissues holding it together while strengthening the muscles surrounding it. And that's why abdominal training is trickier than simple acts of crunching and uncrunching.

The key to a successful crunch is to elevate your torso without rounding your lower back excessively. It helps to try it first when standing:

Stand in an athletic posture—your feet shoulder-width apart, your knees bent slightly—and place one hand on your midsection and one on your lower back. Now crunch your abs down a bit. As you feel your abdominal muscles contracting with one hand, you'll feel your back rounding with the other—that is, you'll feel your spine shifting out of its natural arch.

Try to find a crunching motion that creates the most intense pressure on your abdominal muscles with the least movement in your lower back. That's the sweet spot of abdominal training.

As you get better at this, you should find that you feel the contraction lower in your abdominal wall than you do when you crunch the conventional way, on the floor.

Once you have the sweet spot, try holding it for five breaths. Breathe as deeply as you can without losing the contraction. It won't be easy, but it is useful to teach your midsection muscles to hold this position. You're creating a belt of support to protect your spine under all conditions. If you have to release a contraction every time you breathe, you're putting your spine in jeopardy between breaths.

THE EXERCISES

✳ Swiss-ball crunch

USED IN: Break-In; Fat-Loss I and III; Hypertrophy I, II, and III; Strength I and II

SETUP: Lie on your back on a Swiss ball so your head is level with or slightly lower than your hips. You want your feet flat on the floor and spread apart for balance. Keep your glutes and hamstrings tight. Cross your hands across your chest.

LIFTING: Use your abs to pull your upper torso up as high as it'll go.

LOWERING: Slowly lower yourself to the starting position.

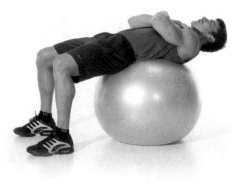

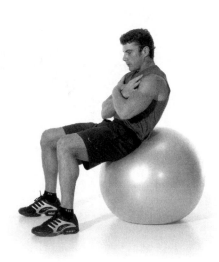

Variations

✳ **Weighted Swiss-ball crunch**

SAME AS ABOVE, EXCEPT . . . When you can do the designated repetitions, using your own body weight, it's time to add some extra resistance. It's up to you when to start doing this—for example, the Break-In program calls for sets of twenty reps on the Swiss-ball crunch. If you know you can do twenty easily, you can start using extra weight from the first set of the first program. As shown in the photos, the easiest way to add weight is to hold a weight plate across your chest. You can also hold one above you at arm's length. Or, to make it really, really challenging, try holding two dumbbells above you at arm's length. Some even hold the plate behind their heads (this version was used by Mark Verstegen* in *Core Performance*). It's your choice.

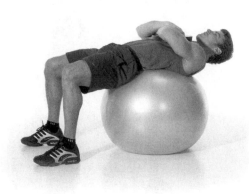
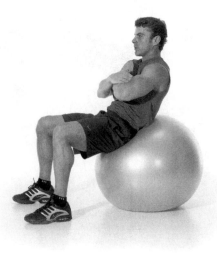

✴ Swiss-ball crunch with medicine-ball throw

USED IN: Strength III

SAME AS ABOVE, EXCEPT . . . Grab a medicine ball, and either have a partner standing a few feet in front of you or set up near a wall that can absorb some good whacks from a weighted ball. (If you're doing this in a gym, you probably want to ask permission before you start flinging away. For example, some people would consider it rude to hammer a ball against a wall when there's a yoga class on the other side.) Hold the ball back behind your head with straight arms, and as you rise, fire the ball to your training partner or against the wall.

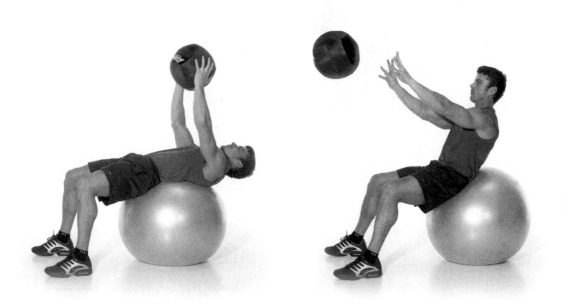

✳ Reverse crunch

USED IN: Break-In; Hypertrophy I

SETUP: Lie on your back on the floor with your arms at your sides, palms-down, and your hips and knees bent 90 degrees. Your thighs are perpendicular to the floor and your lower legs are parallel to it.

LIFTING: Contract your ab muscles as you pull your thighs up toward your chest. The action is in your hips; if your pelvis were a pitcher of water (get your mind out of the gutter), you would be tilting it here, as if pouring the water into a glass.

LOWERING: Slowly lower your legs to the starting position.

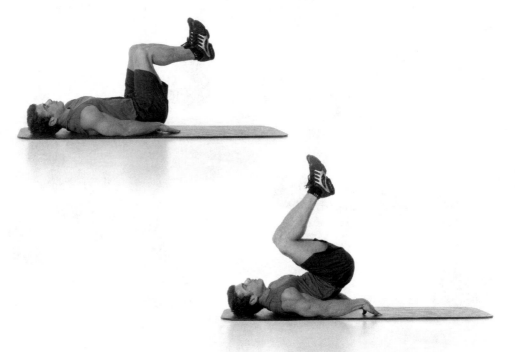

Variation

✳ Incline reverse crunch *(not shown)*

USED IN: Hypertrophy II; Strength I

SAME AS ABOVE, EXCEPT . . . Lie on a slant board, with your hips lower than your head. Grab on to whatever is available to hold your body in place, and do the exercise as described. The stronger you get, the higher the angle you should use.

✳ Swiss-ball lateral roll

USED IN: Fat-Loss I

SETUP: Grab a broomstick and position yourself with your shoulders across a Swiss ball. Hold the broomstick across your upper chest with your arms spread wide. Tighten your glutes and hamstrings and keep your hips high throughout the movement. You want a straight line from your shoulders to your knees; the biggest challenge of the exercise is keeping that alignment as your balance changes.

ACTION: Roll as far as you can to the left, so all your weight is supported by your right shoulder on the ball. Then roll as far as you can to the right. That's one rep.

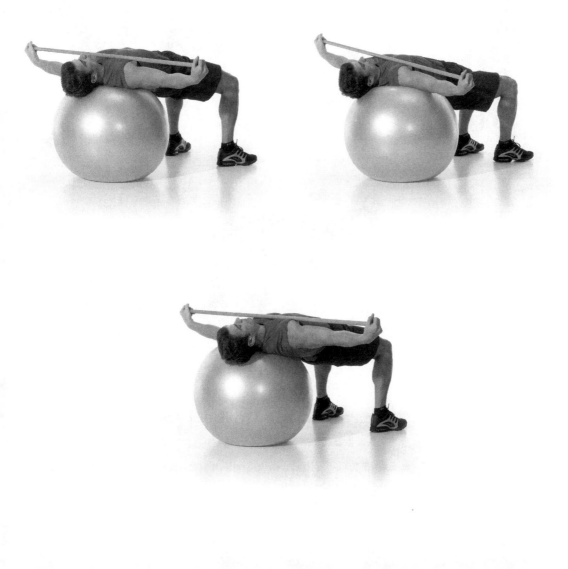

✳ Upper-body Russian twist

USED IN: Fat-Loss II; Hypertrophy II

SETUP: Lie on your back on a Swiss ball with your body in a straight line from chest to knees. Hold your arms straight up from your chest, palms together.

LOWERING: Roll on your shoulders as far as you can to your right, keeping your butt and hamstrings tight and your hips as high as possible.

LIFTING: Roll back as far as you can to your left. That's one rep.

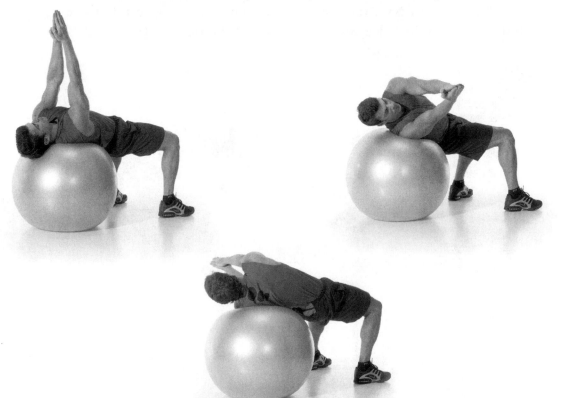

Variation

✳ Dumbbell upper-body Russian twist *(not shown)*

USED IN: Strength II

SAME AS ABOVE, EXCEPT . . . Hold a dumbbell in your hands, one hand on each end as if it were an accordion.

✳ Lower-body Russian twist

USED IN: Fat-Loss II; Strength I

SETUP: Lie on your back on the floor, your arms straight out to your sides, palms-down. Your legs are straight and straight up from your hips.

LOWERING: Lower your legs to your left, keeping them straight and together, going as far as you can without strain.

LIFTING: Lift them straight back along the same path, and continue lowering them to your right side. That's one rep.

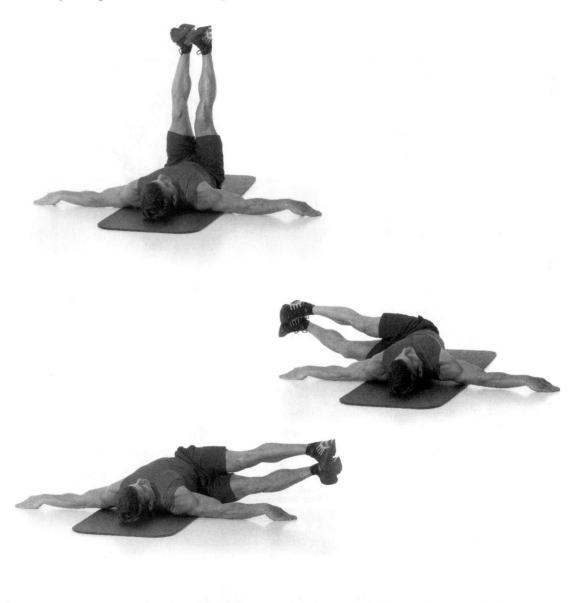

✳ Hanging leg raise

USED IN: Fat-Loss III; Strength II and III

SETUP: Grab a chin-up bar overhand, and hang with your legs together and knees bent. You want your thighs in front of your body somewhat at the start of the lift, just far enough to flatten your lower back. In other words, you want to start the lift with your abdominal muscles already tight and engaged.

LIFTING: Pull your knees up to your chest, rounding your lower back.

LOWERING: Slowly lower them to the starting point, never allowing your abs to disengage or your lower back to arch.

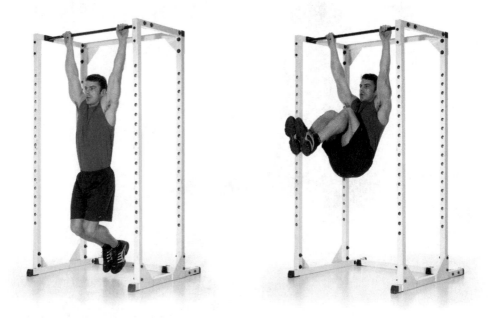

Variations

Not many guys can do high reps, but a few modifications can make it easier. Many gyms now have elbow straps called AbOrigiOnals, which help support your weight and allow more reps (even if they are a crime against spell-checking software). Some people use a device called a captain's chair (it's often part of an apparatus that includes parallel bars for dips), which has elbow rests and a back support. The elbow rests are cool, but the back support is kind of a problem, since it discourages you from rounding your back at the end. That puts a lot more emphasis on the hip flexors and limits the action of your abdominals, which you're trying to target.

✳ **Woodchop**

USED IN: Hypertrophy III; Strength III

SETUP: Attach a rope handle to a high cable pulley; it's easiest to use one inside a cable-crossover station. Stand sideways to the weight stack so your right shoulder faces the weight stack. Grab the rope with both hands and stand far enough away so you have full tension in the cable with your arms straight. Your left arm is reaching across your chest at this point. You want your lower body in an athletic posture—feet shoulder-width apart, knees bent slightly, lower back in its natural arch—and your head turned so your eyes are on your hands, up and to your right.

LIFTING: Pull the rope down and across your body, to just outside your left knee. Your eyes should follow your hands. This is a fast, powerful motion.

LOWERING: Return the cable to the starting position. Finish your reps and then switch sides, pulling to your right.

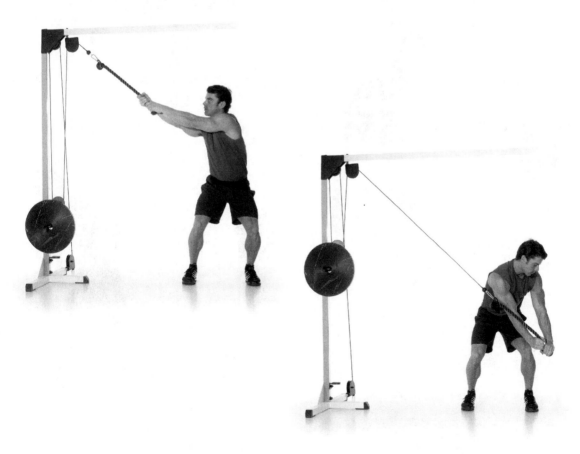

Variation

✳ Reverse woodchop

USED IN: Strength III

SAME AS ABOVE, EXCEPT . . . The rope is on the low pulley, so your hands start just outside your right knee, and you pull up and out so the rope goes past and above your left shoulder. Again, follow your hands with your eyes, and make the motion fast and powerful.

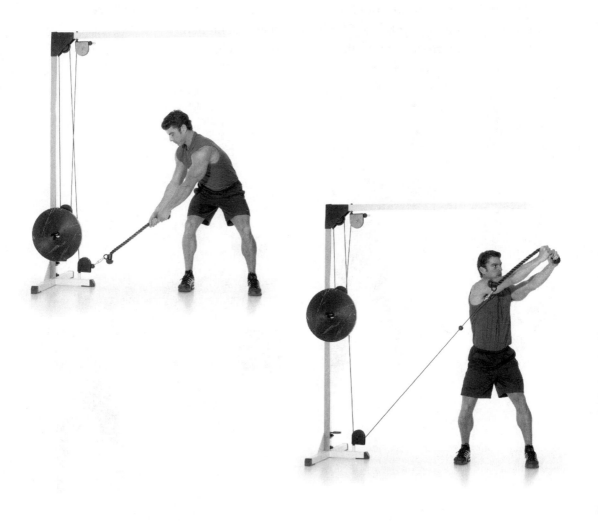

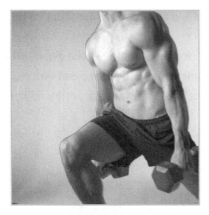

14

Combo Moves

Sports, as I've emphasized in the previous chapters, rarely involve single movement patterns in one particular plane of motion. So even though football players train with the bench press, and tend to be damned good at it, there's nothing in football that precisely mirrors a bench press. Or a squat. Or a deadlift.

That's why most strength coaches have their athletes perform combination moves from time to time. These moves, in some ways, are oddities. On the one hand, they should more closely resemble real-life athletic movements, which involve a collection of actions that require the use of more muscle groups in coordinated action. But then again, there's nothing in sports that resembles a Romanian deadlift/row. So, while you improve coordination somewhat with these exercises, it isn't necessarily coordination that will translate directly to success on the field or court.

Combo moves are harder, though. And harder, as I may have mentioned, is often better. Harder work creates a higher level of stress, which will translate to improved fat loss, as I explain in Chapter 18. That's why you see many combo moves in Alwyn's Fat-Loss programs. Because they force you to involve more muscle mass in each exercise, they'll help you build more of your favorite biologically active tissue. That's why you also see them in Alwyn's Hypertrophy workouts.

Finally, they're simply different from what most people are doing in the gym—all people, really—and it's fun to know you're doing something that's above and beyond the standard-issue, cookie-cutter programs the meatheads and mooks are grinding through.

THE EXERCISES

✳ Romanian deadlift/bent-over row

COMBINES: deadlift, pull

USED IN: Fat-Loss II

SETUP: Load a barbell with a weight you're pretty sure you can row for the designated number of reps. Grab it with an overhand grip just outside shoulder width. Hold it at arm's length in front of your thighs, your knees bent slightly.

LOWERING: Bend at the hips, keeping your knees bent slightly, until the bar is just below your knees and your torso is nearly parallel to the floor, with your lower back in its natural arch.

LIFTING: Pull the bar to your abdomen, as in a bent-over row.

LOWERING: Lower the bar to arm's length again.

LIFTING: Now straighten your hips, as in a Romanian deadlift. That's one rep.

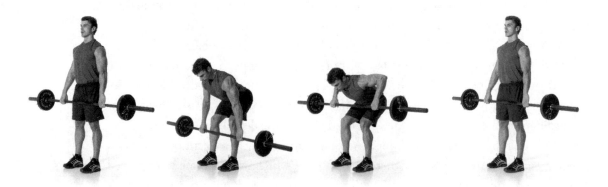

✳ High pull

COMBINES: deadlift, pull

USED IN: Hypertrophy I

SETUP: Load a barbell with a weight you would use in a shoulder press. Grab it with an overhand grip just outside shoulder width, and hold it in front of your thighs.

LOWERING: Bend your knees and bend forward slightly at the hips, as if you were preparing to jump. The bar stays in contact with your thighs as it slides down a few inches.

LIFTING: Now you're going to do a facsimile of a jump, as you simultaneously come up on your toes and straighten your knees and hips. In the same motion, pull the bar up to your chest. Try to increase the speed and fluidity of the movement in subsequent workouts; it really should feel like jumping, only with a bar in your hands.

DON'T LET THIS HAPPEN TO YOU: Our friend Charles Staley, a strength coach in Phoenix, once told me a story that should serve as a caution for everyone who enjoys and gets good at high pulls. He once pulled so hard that he hit himself in the chin with the bar. When he came to, he was flat on his back, with blood flowing from his mouth. The lesson: Take it easy with lighter weights. I've popped myself in the chin a couple of times. I wasn't hurt, but the experience made me remember Staley's knock-out experience.

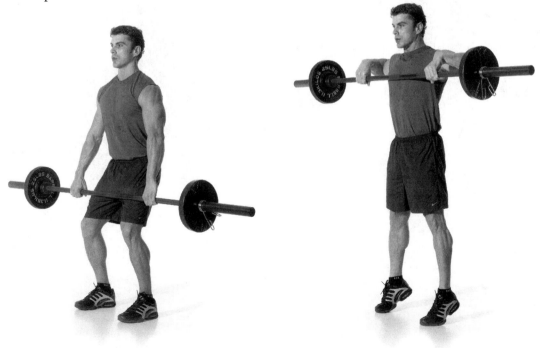

✳ Jefferson lunge

COMBINES: deadlift, lunge

USED IN: Hypertrophy III

SETUP: Load a barbell with a weight that you might use in a dynamic lunge. (Remember, if the workout calls for eight reps, that means eight with *each leg,* or sixteen total per set.) Set your legs in a split-squat position, with your weaker leg (probably your left) in front and the bar directly beneath your torso. Reach down and grab it with an overhand grip just outside shoulder width. Straighten your legs as you rise up as high as you can without endangering your future heirs.

LOWERING: Go down as you normally would in a lunge or split squat, with your forward knee bent about 90 degrees and your rear knee almost touching the floor.

LIFTING: Rise back to the starting position. That's one rep. Do the designated reps, switch legs, and repeat to finish the set.

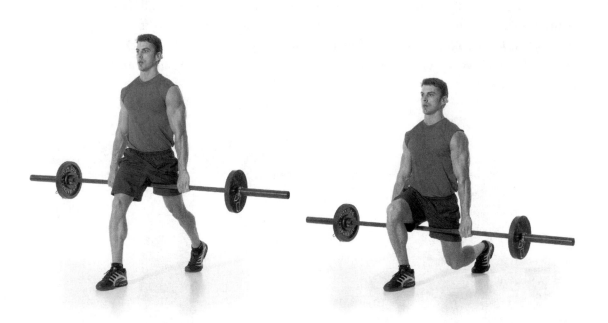

✳ Split good morning

COMBINES: deadlift, lunge

USED IN: Hypertrophy III

SETUP: Load an Olympic bar with a weight that's a bit lighter than the one you used for the Bulgarian split deadlifts, with which you're alternating this exercise. (Alternating sets are explained in Chapter 18 on page 212.) If you have to do both exercises with one barbell, decide on the weight you'll use for both exercises before you begin, and make sure you can easily slide a couple of plates off the barbell so you can go directly to this exercise with no more than the designated rest between exercises. Get a step from the aerobics studio; you want it about four to six inches off the floor. Lift the bar past your head to your traps, and hold it as you would for a squat or good morning. Finally, place one foot (probably your left) flat on the step, and the other about eighteen to twenty-four inches behind it (measured from front heel to rear toe). Your front knee should be bent, your rear leg straight, and your torso upright, with your back naturally arched.

LOWERING: Bend forward at the hips until your torso is nearly parallel to the floor, or until your hamstrings threaten to file a restraining order. (In other words, don't lower yourself to the point of pain.)

LIFTING: Straighten your torso to the starting position. That's one rep. Do all the designated reps with this leg forward, then switch legs and repeat.

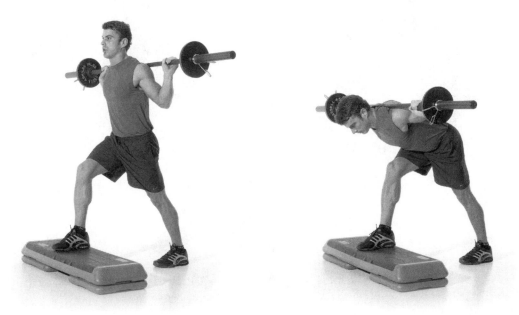

✳ Bulgarian split squat with overhead press

COMBINES: lunge, pull, push

USED IN: Fat-Loss II

SETUP: Grab a pair of dumbbells that you think you can use for shoulder presses for the designated reps. (Remember to multiply by two, since you're going to do all the reps with each leg forward to complete a set.) Stand with your legs split, the top of your rear foot resting on a bench. (Again, start with your weaker leg, probably your left, in front.) Hold the dumbbells with straight arms, your palms facing your sides.

LOWERING: As you lower your torso until your front knee is bent to about 90 degrees, "clean" the dumbbells to your shoulders (a clean is sort of a fast curl).

LIFTING: Press the weights overhead, then lower them to your shoulders. Lift your torso back to the starting position, then lower the dumbbells back to your sides. That's one rep. Do all the designated reps with this leg forward, then switch legs and repeat.

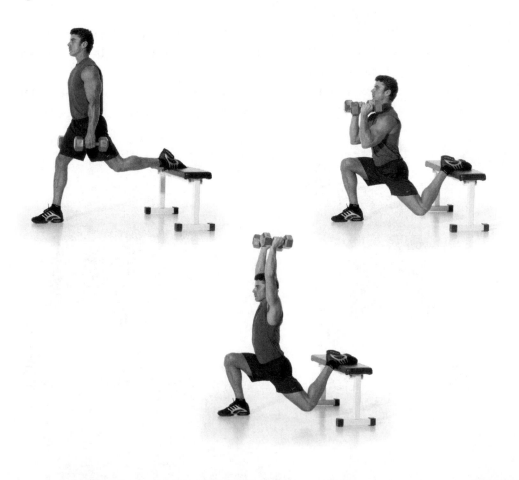

✳ Walking lunge with side bend

COMBINES: lunge, twist

USED IN: Fat-Loss III

SETUP: Grab a pair of dumbbells and hold them at your sides as you stand with your feet hip-width apart, and as much walking room in front of you as possible.

LOWERING: Take a lunge-step forward with your left leg (start the next set with your right leg, if you can remember; no big deal if you can't). As you lower yourself to the point at which your front knee is bent to about 90 degrees and your rear knee is near the floor, bend to your left side.

LIFTING: Straighten your torso as you rise to the starting position, and immediately go into a forward lunge-step with your right leg and bend to your right. Continue lunging until you've completed the set; each lunge-step-and-lean counts as one rep, so in a twenty-rep set, you'll do ten with each leg.

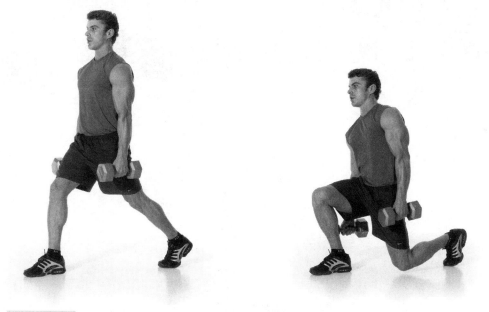

Variation

✳ Rotational lunge *(not shown)*

USED IN: Fat-Loss I

SAME AS ABOVE, EXCEPT . . . As you lunge forward with your left leg, rotate your torso to the left. Then rotate your torso to the right as you lunge with your right leg.

✳ T-push-up

COMBINES: push, twist

USED IN: Fat-Loss II

SETUP: Get down on the floor, into push-up position.

LOWERING: Lower your chest to the floor.

LIFTING: Push yourself up, then twist to your right side, lifting your right arm so it's perpendicular to the floor and forms a straight line with your torso and left arm. Your eyes should follow your hand, so you're looking up in this top position. That's one rep. Now return to the starting position, then repeat, twisting to your left. That's your second rep. If the set calls for eight, you'll do four twists to each side.

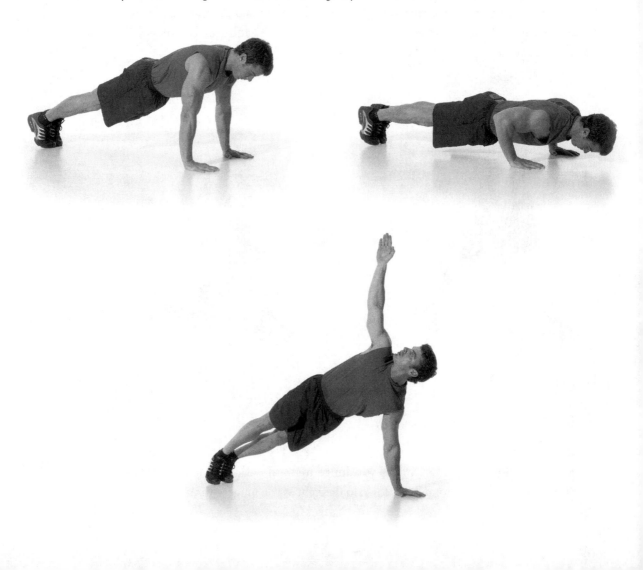

ADDING WEIGHTS: As soon as you can, use a dumbbell, preferably one with hexagonal edges (round ones are okay, but they do add a balance challenge, especially when you get to the point at which you can do this with two dumbbells).

One dumbbell: Get into push-up position with the weight in your right hand. Now as you twist to the right, you'll be lifting a weight, increasing the challenge. Do half the designated reps with your right hand, then repeat with the weight in your left.

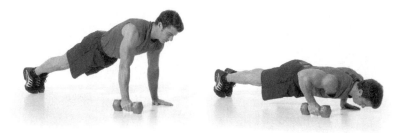

Two dumbbells: Now you'll start in push-up position with a dumbbell in each hand (if they aren't hexagonal, you're doing a circus trick at this point). Alternate to the right and left with each repetition.

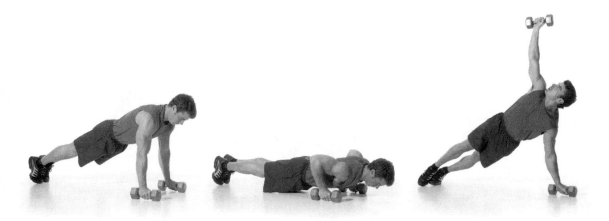

✳ Deadlift shrug *(not shown)*

COMBINES: deadlift, pull

USED IN: Hypertrophy I

SET-UP: Load a barbell and set up as you would for a deadlift, with your feet shoulder-width apart, your hands just outside your legs and gripping the bar over-hand, your back in its natural arch, and your shoulders over the bar.

LIFTING: Pull the bar straight up along your legs, as you would in a deadlift. But instead of stopping when your torso is straight, continue pulling with your shoulders, using a shrugging motion. Keep your arms straight. As you get better at it and develop more speed on the lift, you can come up on your toes if you want.

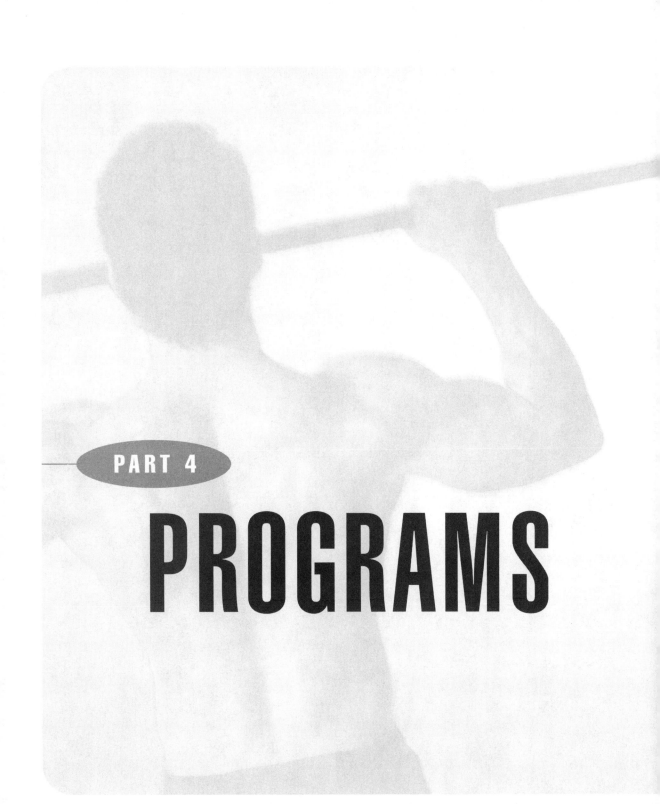

PART 4

PROGRAMS

15

How to Choose the Right Program for You

A<small>LL</small> <small>RIGHT</small>, *now* it's time to train. And it only took me fourteen chapters to get here. (My wife would tell you that's pretty good, by my standards.)

Alwyn has created three training programs, one each for fat loss, hypertrophy (the fancy word for "muscle growth"), and pure strength.

Each program has three phases. Each phase is meant to stand on its own as a multi-week program, but the phases also build on one another. Thus, the gains you make in Phase 1 prepare you for Phase 2, and Phase 2 prepares you for Phase 3. You can do all three phases of any program consecutively, and that's fine.

But the real beauty of Alwyn's vision here—the reason this book is different from any other we've seen—is that the programs can be broken down into modular parts for you to mix and match, based on your shifting goals and preferences.

Everyone will start with the Break-In program, which I'll show and explain in Chapter 17. But after that, you've got the chance to create an individualized training system that you can follow for months or even years without having to look elsewhere for new routines and challenges.

Let's look at four lifters, and how each would put together his own system from Alwyn's programs. For the sake of simplicity, I'm going to assume each lifter starts in the first week of January.

LIFTER #1: THE ETERNAL BEGINNER

Let's say you're thirty-five. You've never followed a program for more than a couple of months. You'll join a gym in January, or renew your membership to the gym you joined the previous January, and you'll do pretty well until you find yourself losing the spark around Valentine's Day. You go through the motions for a few more weeks, but by St. Patrick's Day you're running on fumes. Since you've made no gains since late January, your motivation is sapped.

The great thing about you is that your body has made very few adaptations to exercise. That means virtually everything you try is going to produce visceral, measurable, visual results. You'll feel better, you'll see your strength improving every week, and you'll be able to see it all working when you look in a mirror. Others will see it, too.

Your plan:

Weeks 1–4: Break-In program

Two workouts a week for four weeks.

Week 5: Off

Seriously, you'll take a breather this week. Your body has made some improvements in strength and muscle size. Even though those changes aren't dramatic, your body is still going through a remodeling process. So here you'll give it a week to catch up. If your muscle strength is getting ahead of your tendon strength, we'll slow it down a bit and let everything recover completely. (Connective tissues have a smaller blood supply than muscle fibers, so their recovery is always compromised somewhat compared to your muscles'.)

There's also a psychological reason for taking that time off: Your body is probably just starting to "get" the routine. You're getting good at it. A couple more workouts, and you'll hit a peak with these exercises, in this order. And we absolutely do not want you to peak on anything. We want you to leave a little in the tank. We want you to wish you were at the gym, finishing what you started, throughout the week you're not there. Believe me, wishing you could go to the gym when you can't is a hundred times better than wishing you weren't there when you could be.

Weeks 6–9: Fat-Loss I

Three workouts a week for four weeks.

Week 10: Off

Same reasons, except now you've made some serious improvements—less fat, certainly, and probably some gains in muscle size and strength. (Beginners have that magical ability to improve in both directions at once.) You've also increased your workload from ten exercise sets twice a week to eighteen sets three times a week. And you've done that for four weeks, using heavier weights every week, with shorter rest periods in between sets.

Weeks 11–14: Fat-Loss II

Three workouts a week for four weeks.

Week 15: Off

The exercise volume in Fat-Loss II is the same as before—eighteen sets, three times a week—but the loads are heavier (in the final workouts of Fat-Loss II, you do sets of eight reps, with heavier weights than you've used so far), and the rest periods are even shorter. Big gains? Oh, yes. The mirror alone should show a very different image by this point, four months into the program. If you're following the diet suggestions in Part 5, you've probably lost a couple of inches off your waist. You feel more "toned" (much as I hate to use that word) from shoulders to calves, with your muscles harder to the touch, and the contours of all your muscle groups more pronounced.

That's why it's the perfect time to take another break here. We want you to be aware that adaptations like these come with a price; you can pay the price up front, by giving your body a chance to recover fully, or you can pay it weeks or months down the road, with an injury.

Weeks 16–23: Hypertrophy I

Three workouts a week for eight weeks.

Week 24: Off

I'll explain the shock and awe of Alwyn's first Hypertrophy program in Chapter 19. Here, I'll simply note that it involves shifting around between three set-and-rep configurations for the major exercises: five sets of five reps, three sets of fifteen, four sets of ten. That's a lot more volume, and much heavier weights in some of the workouts. Take a week to recover, or perhaps even two if you feel beaten up here.

Weeks 25–32: Hypertrophy II

Three workouts a week for eight weeks.

Week 33: Off

The swings in Hypertrophy II are even more extreme: six sets of three, on up to two sets of twenty-five. You'll have fun, and you'll see gains you didn't think your body was capable of making, but you'll need this break. Seriously.

Weeks 34–39: Strength I

Three workouts a week for five weeks, with one workout in the sixth week.

Week 40: Off

You're also taking most of Week 39 off, so this is nearly a two-week break. But given the fact that you'll have just done the most aggressive program yet, lifting the heaviest weights you've ever lifted, your shoulders, knees, and elbows will be very happy to have this break.

Weeks 41–46: Strength II

Three workouts a week for five weeks, with one workout in the sixth week.

Week 47: Off

You're also taking most of Week 46 off, so this is nearly a two-week break. You need the time off for the reasons I mentioned earlier, along with the fact that you're about to do the most aggressive and grueling workout in the entire program. So you're recovering and mustering energy at the same time.

Weeks 48–51: Fat-Loss III

Three workouts a week for four weeks.

Week 52: Off

If you started the program the first week in January, you're so much bigger, stronger, and leaner by Christmas that your friends and family may not recognize you. So go reintroduce yourself to them.

LIFTER #2: THE GUY WHO CONSIDERS "SKINNY" AN INSULT

Let's say you're twenty-two, six feet tall, 160 pounds. Maybe you can see your abs, but to you it's no badge of honor, considering you can also count your ribs by looking in a mirror . . . from fifty feet away. I'm going to assume you're an intermediate lifter, perhaps with a history of bouncing around from program to program (like, every time a new issue of *Flex* hits the newsstand). You're embarrassed to say how many sets of biceps curls you do in an average week, despite the fact that your biceps stopped growing in your freshman year of college.

Weeks 1–4: Break-In program

Three workouts a week for three weeks, with the tenth and final workout on the first training day of the fourth week. Take the rest of the week off.

Weeks 5–10: Hypertrophy I

Four workouts a week for six weeks.

Week 11: Off

Seem absurd to take a week off, when you're just getting started? Yes, except I have a sneaking hunch you've been doing a lot of "bonus" work during the initial programs. Like, ten extra sets of curls, extensions, and lateral raises after each workout? Fine; admitting you have a problem is the first step toward recovery. This week is for that recovery.

Weeks 12–19: Hypertrophy II

Three workouts a week for eight weeks.

Weeks 20–21: Off

Because I know you really worked out five times a week for the past two months.

Weeks 22–25: Strength I

Four workouts a week for four weeks.

Week 26: Off

At least this time I'm pretty sure you didn't sneak in any extra workouts. And I'll bet that wave-loading those squats made you look forward to this break. (The phrase "wave-loading" will make sense when you read Chapter 20.)

Weeks 27–30: Strength II

Four workouts a week for four weeks.

Week 31: Off

Thought it looked easy, didn't you? But then you actually tried those quarter-squats in Strength II, and you realized they aren't the fun kind, the ones where you think you're Iron Man because you're doing these instead of full squats. You learned that these quarter-squats are the ones where you use more than 100 percent of your one-rep max and descend only partway on purpose. Whole different sensation.

Weeks 32–37: Hypertrophy III

Four workouts a week for six weeks.

Week 38: Off

By now you're with the program, and not even tempted to sneak in those extra-credit sets. Still, after six weeks of slamming your body every which way, including loose, you'll be happy for this little interlude.

Weeks 39–42: Strength III

Four workouts a week for four weeks.

Weeks 43–44: Off

You won't argue.

Weeks 45–50: Fat-Loss II and Fat-Loss III

Four workouts a week for three weeks on each program, with no break in between.

Week 51–52: Off

Now go show off that bigger, stronger, and still-lean (thanks to those six weeks of Fat-Loss workouts at the end) physique of yours.

LIFTER #3: A MAN OF CONSTANT OBLIGATION

You're twenty-nine, your job demands your brain, and your young children demand your energy. All you have left is your body, which you love to challenge with hard workouts and heavy weights. But workouts feel more like a luxury these days, and you find yourself getting to the gym erratically—sometimes four times a week, sometimes . . . almost once. And yet this is your favorite activity that doesn't bring in revenue for your company or improve the quality of life for your family.

I'm going to propose something very radical: You're going to train just twice a week but forbid yourself to skip either of those two workouts. The way Alwyn's system is set up, you can do these workouts on consecutive days if you have to, or separated by four or five days if that's your only choice. The one absolute is that you're going to squeeze in two workouts a week. If you can do more, fine; the system allows for you to do that, as long as you keep alternating the workouts in Alwyn's designated order.

Also, I'm assuming you're an intermediate-to-advanced lifter, perhaps a former athlete who's had some coaching. But, because of your erratic schedule (and some late-night stress-relief eating, thanks to the kids' shaky sleep-wake cycles), you've put on a few pounds around the middle. Your brain may remember how to do the exercises, but your body will nonetheless struggle with executing them at first.

Weeks 1–3: Break-In program

Two workouts a week for three weeks.

Week 4: Off

Weeks 5–8: Fat-Loss II

Two workouts a week for four weeks. (You skipped Fat-Loss I because you've already done similar sets and reps, and similar exercises, in the Break-In program.)

Week 9: Off

Weeks 10–15: Hypertrophy I

Two workouts a week for six weeks. The charts indicate that you should perform a total of twenty-four workouts. But you're stopping at twelve, since your body will probably make most of the potential adaptations after six weeks. And even if it doesn't, six weeks is long enough for this program.

Week 16: Off

Weeks 17–24: Strength I

Two workouts a week for eight weeks. This program has four workouts, so it'll take you two weeks to do each of them, and eight weeks to cycle through each four times.

Weeks 25–26: Off

Perfect time for a summer vacation.

Weeks 27–34: Strength II

Two workouts a week for eight weeks. (Same as Strength I.)

Week 35: Off

Weeks 36–43: Strength III

Two workouts a week for eight weeks. (Same as Strength I and II.)

Week 44: Off

Weeks 45–50: Fat-Loss III

Two workouts a week for six weeks. No, you aren't doing this because you're fat. You're doing it to give your muscles some new stimulation—high-rep sets following Strength programs will have that effect.

Weeks 51–52: Off

You not only need a break, you've earned it.

LIFTER #4: SERIOUS ABOUT LIFTING, BUT SERIOUSLY OVERWEIGHT

You're forty-five, and you've been lifting since the beginning of time. Since you were fifteen, anyway. In fact, you were the bench-press champion of your college fraternity four consecutive years, and you seriously considered flunking a couple of classes your final semester so you could return to campus and win it again. You're still a strong guy, although no one could tell by looking at you.

Yes, you still hit the gym three or four times a week, but most of your "program" involves sitting on a bench, working on your biceps, triceps, delts, and pecs.

So, even though your arms and chest and shoulders are bigger than ever, so is your gut. And your legs seem smaller by comparison with every passing year.

Let's be frank: About three-quarters of the work you need to do to get back in shape will take place outside the gym. You'll need to read Part 5 carefully, and adopt an every-waking-hour diet plan that gives you enough energy to train and enough food to kill hunger pangs but also allows you to lose fat safely and steadily.

In the gym, you also need to change your approach. You have a world of potential, since you already know how to lift and are in the habit. But you also have one significant handicap: Your body has already adapted to many of the programs we could throw your way. To use a rather strange metaphor in this context, all the low-hanging fruit has been plucked.

That would ordinarily be a problem. But you're lucky: You have Alwyn Cosgrove on your side. Here's how to use Alwyn's *New Rules* programs for your transformation.

Weeks 1–4: Break-In program

Start on the Intermediate plan, with total-body workouts three days a week. But we want you to do something that we haven't suggested for the others: After each of these workouts, we want you to do the "Metabolic Overdrive" interval program, shown in Chapter 7. In Week 4, you'll only lift once, but you can do intervals three times.

Weeks 5–8: Fat-Loss II

Three workouts a week for four weeks. Continue with the intervals, cranking up the intensity as described in Chapter 7.

Week 9: Off

Take a break from everything here, including the intervals.

Weeks 10–13: Fat-Loss III

Three workouts a week for four weeks. Continue with the intervals, cranking up the intensity as described.

Week 14: Off

Lay off the weights but continue with the intervals, reaching peak intensity. This is it for intervals for a while, so make these count. At the end of each session, finish with the warm-up exercises shown in Chapter 5—treat them more as flexibility exercises than true warm-ups. You can also do ab exercises and some light calisthenics if you choose.

Weeks 15–22: Hypertrophy I

Three workouts a week for eight weeks.

Weeks 23–24: Off

Stay active, and eat clean at least 80 percent of the time. ("Clean eating" is described in Chapter 22.)

Weeks 25–32: Hypertrophy III

Three workouts a week for eight weeks.

Week 33: Off

If you want to hit the gym this week, resume the interval program, starting at the beginning. Don't push yourself here; the goal is to get your body used to it again.

Weeks 34–39: Strength I

Three workouts a week for the first five weeks, and one workout in the sixth week. (Strength I has four workouts, and you want to do each four times. So the sixteenth workout will fall on the first gym day of the sixth week.) Continue with the intervals as before.

Week 40: Off

This is really close to a two-week break from the weights. Continue with the intervals, cranking up the intensity as you did earlier in the year.

Weeks 41–46: Strength II

Three workouts a week for the first five weeks, and one workout in the sixth week. Use the balance of the sixth week to peak on your intervals.

Weeks 47–50: Fat-Loss I

Three workouts a week for four weeks. Now, after eleven months of progressively harder work, you're going to downshift. It's like an athlete's taper before the biggest event of his competitive season: You'll finish the year with higher reps, basic exercises, and a break from the heaviest weights, as well as the peak-intensity intervals.

Here's the real beauty of it: Since you haven't done high-rep sets for months at this point, it'll be something new for your body. So will the reduced workload. As your body starts to "catch up," muscles will become more visible, even as the tightness that accrues from steady, hard training starts to fade away. You'll feel better and look better.

Another benefit of the taper is that it helps reduce pre-holiday stress while giving you a body that's better rested and recovered for next year's programs.

Weeks 51–52: Off

Lather, Rinse . . . Repeat?

In the four examples, you'll notice that the lifters never repeat specific workouts. Which brings up a logical question: Should workouts ever be repeated? Alwyn says it's okay to re-peat, as long as you put at least twelve weeks in between. In other words, it's fine to start the year with a Fat-Loss program, move on to Hypertrophy programs, and then shift back to the original Fat-Loss program to get a little leaner for summer. Just follow the twelve-week rule, and the programs should work fine the second time around.

16

Charting Your Progress

STARTING IN CHAPTER 17, you're going to see a series of workout charts telling you the exercises to do for each phase of each program, as well as the number of sets and repetitions, the amount of time you should rest between sets, and even the speed at which you should perform your repetitions.

The best way to keep track of all that is with a system of workout charts. On page 203, you'll see a blank chart that will work for any of Alwyn's *New Rules* workouts. You just need to copy it, and then fill in the appropriate words and numbers in the appropriate columns. (A sample chart appears on page 204.)

The New Rules of Lifting
Program:
Workout:

Exercise	Sets	Reps	Set 1	Set 2	Set 3	Set 4	Set 5	Set 6	Tempo	Rest
Workout 1										
Workout 2										
Workout 3										
Workout 4										
Workout 1										
Workout 2										
Workout 3										
Workout 4										
Workout 1										
Workout 2										
Workout 3										
Workout 4										
Workout 1										
Workout 2										
Workout 3										
Workout 4										
Workout 1										
Workout 2										
Workout 3										
Workout 4										
Workout 1										
Workout 2										
Workout 3										
Workout 4										

Notes: _____

_____

_____

SAMPLE

The New Rules of Lifting
Program: Fat-Loss I
Workout: A

Exercise	Sets	Reps	Set 1	Set 2	Set 3	Set 4	Set 5	Set 6	Tempo	Rest
Alternating sets										
Barbell squat									Normal	75
Workout 1	3	15	65/15	75/15	85/13					
Workout 2	3	15	75/15	85/15	95/11					
Workout 3										
Workout 4										
Cable seated row to waist									Normal	75
Workout 1	3	15	40/15	45/15	50/15					
Workout 2	3	15	50/15	55/15	60/14					
Workout 3										
Workout 4										
Alternating sets										
Supine hip extension (body weight)									Normal	75
Workout 1	3	15	15	14	12					
Workout 2	3	15	15	15	15					
Workout 3										
Workout 4										
Dumbbell push press									Normal	75
Workout 1	3	15	25/15	30/14	30/12					
Workout 2	3	15	30/15	35/13	35/11					
Workout 3										
Workout 4										
Alternating sets										
Dumbbell rotational lunge									Normal	75
Workout 1	3	15	10/15	15/15	15/11					
Workout 2	3	15	15/15	20/15	20/12					
Workout 3										
Workout 4										
Swiss-ball crunch (body weight)									Normal	75
Workout 1	3	15	15	15	13					
Workout 2	3	15	15	15	14					
Workout 3										
Workout 4										

Notes: _____

_____

_____

. . .

A few questions you may have:

✳   **Why are there blank spaces between pairs of exercises?**
Alwyn uses alternating sets in many of his programs. The lines allow you to write that, or any other instructions you may need there. (Don't worry if you don't know what an alternating set is yet; all terms and instructions are fully explained in the workout chapters.)

✳   **What do the numbers under "Set 1," "Set 2," and "Set 3" mean?**
The first number is the amount of weight you use on that set. The second is the number of repetitions you complete. So "40/15" means you did fifteen reps with forty pounds.

✳   **How come the lifter in this sample did fewer than fifteen reps on some sets?**
When you get into the gym and start doing these programs, you'll find that you sometimes underestimate how much weight you can use. If you get fifteen reps on all three sets with a weight, you can be pretty sure you undershot your strength potential on that exercise. But most of us go the other direction. We choose a weight that's a bit too heavy to get all the reps on all three sets, and that's why this lifter falls short on some sets. There's no problem with falling short—you have to try a weight before you can know whether it's too light or too heavy.

Another factor is exhaustion. You may have chosen the right weight, but then run out of gas before the end of the set.

✳   **Should I use the weights shown in this sample as my ideal starting weights?**
No. You have to estimate your own starting weights, using trial and error. There's no way to get around it. I've met personal trainers who were phenomenally good at figuring out their clients' starting weights. Alwyn is among them. Maybe it's some kind of Jedi mind trick. But unless you have one of those trainers, you have to figure it out on your own.

✳   **What does the phrase "body weight" mean in the entries for the Supine hip extension and Swiss-ball crunch?**
That means you do the exercises with your body weight for resistance. You have the option of using a weight on the Swiss-ball crunch, but there's no practical way to add resistance on the Supine hip extension.

If you're doing a combination of body weight and resistance—holding a weight plate across your chest, say—on the Swiss-ball crunch, you can indicate that on your log by using "BW" for body weight. If this sample had chosen that strategy, he might've written "BW/15" for Set 1, meaning he did fifteen reps with his body weight as the only resistance. Then if he added weight for subsequent sets, he could write "10/15" for Set 2, meaning he completed fifteen reps with ten pounds, then "15/12," meaning he ran out of gas after doing twelve reps with fifteen pounds.

✳ **What happens if I need to do a particular workout more than four times?**
Just use a second blank page, and write in "Workout 5" where it says "Workout 1," etc.

✳ **Tempo? What the hell?**
"Tempo" is the speed of your repetitions, your rhythm. When a workout designates "normal" tempo, we assume you'll lift at the speed that feels most natural to you, unless "natural" is a series of spasms and jerks that would get you kicked out of the gym if you didn't have a barbell in your hands.

We expect an average lifter to take two or three seconds to lower a weight, pause for a second, and then take a second to lift it. But your "natural" tempo may be faster or slower than that. It doesn't matter. The key is to know what your normal speed is so you know when you're speeding it up or slowing it down.

There will be times in this program when Alwyn prescribes a specific tempo for you, but I'll explain that when you get to those workouts.

✳ **Won't I look silly carrying these pages around?**
I've been carrying around workout sheets on a clipboard for so many years that I can't remember the last time I worried about someone thinking less of me because of my record-keeping. Frankly, I can't think of any reason why they would. The guys who draw snickers are the ones who think they know what they're doing but don't— the guys who load up a bar with too much weight in the bench-press station, use a spotter to help them complete the lift, and then jump around like they've just won an Olympic medal.

I tend to see two types of lifters using workout logs: the newbies, who're trying to follow programs created by their trainers, and the most serious, goal-oriented intermediate and advanced lifters. Granted, that's still a minority of the gym population. But if there's any "dork factor" involved in following a written program and keeping track of your progress, I'm not aware of it.

17

Break-In Program

Alwyn wants everyone to do this program for at least two weeks before advancing to the regular routines. Yes, that includes you, even if you're so buff you just won your neighborhood's Mr. Cul-de-Sac trophy for the third year in a row.

He says that for two reasons: First, the programs in the following chapters are complex, and you need some amount of muscular endurance to perform them effectively. Second, many lifters today have never actually gone through a basic, balanced, total-body program. Alwyn and I and every other trainer in America can tell you stories about guys who walk into the gym for the first time with programs they ripped out of *Muscle & Fitness* and start off doing fifteen sets of biceps curls and another fifteen sets of triceps extensions.

Hell, look at me: I lifted for a quarter-century before I did my first set of deadlifts and second set of squats. (As I said in Chapter 8, the first set of squats didn't go very well.)

So, no matter your muscle mass, regardless of your reputation, do this Break-In program for four weeks if you're a beginner, and at least two weeks if you're advanced.

Some definitions:

Beginner

I don't necessarily mean a *beginner* beginner—as in, you're really trying to lift for the first time. If you've never lifted for more than a few months without stopping and you haven't been on any program for more than a month, consider yourself a beginner.

Do each of the two workouts once a week, with as much time in between as your schedule allows. (Monday and Thursday is perfect, but if you have to do it more erratically, no sweat. Just make sure there's at least one day between workouts.)

Intermediate

We define an intermediate as a guy who has, at some point, lifted for at least a year without taking a substantial break (longer than two or three weeks). Be smart about this: You know if you've lifted long enough to get the hang of it. You should be able to say you've tried a variety of exercises and have seen measurable progress, both in terms of strength and exercise performance and in what you see in the mirror. Physical changes—bigger muscles, smaller waist—are a pretty good indicator that your body has made some physiological adaptations, and you're thus a true intermediate.

Do each workout four or five times, alternating between the A and B programs, with at least one day of rest in between each. Ideally, you'll do three workouts a week (Monday, Wednesday, Friday, for example) for three weeks. That's nine total workouts, so to make sure you do both workouts an equal number of times, you'd do the tenth and final Break-In workout on Monday of the fourth week. Then you'd take the rest of the fourth week off before diving into one of the other programs.

Alternately, you could do the workouts four times each, ending the program on Monday of the third week.

Advanced

We all think we're advanced, but few of us really are. An advanced lifter should be able to say he's lifted for years without a serious break and that those years were both consecutive and adjacent to the current one.

A test of whether you're truly advanced: If you make all the adjustments you're going to make to a new workout program within two weeks, you're advanced.

Do each workout twice a week for two weeks (two days on, one off, two on, two off) before jumping into the Strength or Hypertrophy programs.

Alternating sets

When two or more exercises appear under the heading "alternating sets," you simply switch back and forth from one exercise to the next, resting in between each set of each exercise, until you've finished all the sets of each exercise.

In Break-In Workout A, the first time you use alternating sets is with static lunges and two-point dumbbell rows. The chart tells you to do two sets of each exercise, with sixty seconds' rest in between.

So you do the first set of lunges, rest sixty seconds, do the first set of rows, rest sixty seconds, do the second set of lunges, rest, do the second set of rows, rest, and then move on to the next pair of exercises.

You'll notice that these exercises include an asterisk telling you to do all the reps (fifteen for each exercise) with each leg or arm. That means you're doing thirty total reps per set of each exercise, since you're doing fifteen with each leg or arm.

Here's the full sequence:

- 15 lunges with one leg
- 15 lunges with the other leg
- Rest
- 15 rows with one arm
- 15 rows with the other arm
- Rest

Repeat the sequence, and move on to the next pair of exercises.

Break-In Workout A				
Exercise	**Sets**	**Reps**	**Tempo**	**Rest**
Squat (p. 96)	2	15	Normal	60
Alternating sets				
Static lunge (p. 123)	2	15*	Normal	60
Two-point dumbbell row with elbow out (p. 158)	2	15*	Normal	60
Alternating sets				
Push-up (p. 135)	2	15	Normal	60
Swiss-ball crunch (p. 169)	2	20	Normal	60
*each leg or arm				

Break-In Workout B

Exercise	Sets	Reps	Tempo	Rest
Deadlift (p. 106)	2	15	Normal	60
Alternating sets				
Step-up (p. 126)	2	15*	Normal	60
Dumbbell one-arm shoulder press (p. 143)	2	15*	Normal	60
Alternating sets				
Close-grip lat pulldown (p. 152)	2	15	Normal	60
Reverse crunch (p. 172)	2	20	Normal	60

*each leg or arm

Fat-Loss Programs

A GUY WHO'S TRYING to burn fat has two enemies in the weight room: efficiency and adaptation. The second is easy enough to understand: Your body adapts to workout routines. That means the longer you do the same thing, the less benefit comes from it. Furthermore, the longer you lift—in terms of months and years—the faster your body adapts to any new workout.

You can give adaptation a more positive spin by looking at it from the other direction: When you give your body something new to try, something for which it hasn't yet developed a strategy to make it easier, your body has to make adjustments.

These adjustments come from a variety of different biological systems. Your muscles and the nerves that make them work have to learn new movements. That could mean more strain on your muscles, creating a greater turnover of the proteins in your muscle fibers (more breaking down, more building up). That by itself could speed up your metabolism, meaning you burn more calories in the hours and perhaps even days following your workout.

Unfamiliar exercises could also provoke a stronger response from your sympathetic nervous system. This is your "fight or flight" stress response—quicker and stronger pulse, tighter sphincter, more sweat, wider air passages. The stress response gets a bad rap, but it's one of your best friends in the gym. It kicks in quickly when you start exercising, releasing adrenaline. Adrenaline (also called epinephrine) opens up your blood vessels. More blood flow means more energy for your muscles, and faster contractions. (I probably should've mentioned this in Chapter 5, when I discussed the importance of warming up. But . . . well, I forgot. Sorry.)

The longer you train with specific exercises, the lower your stress-hormone response to those movements. That's great if you're working to get stronger. You want your body to become more efficient at the exercise, and part of that efficiency is a lower level of stress associated with it.

But if you're trying to lose fat, efficiency is the enemy. You want your body to react with *more* stress. Besides the rush of adrenaline that comes with stress, making harder work possible, another hormone works to your advantage: cortisol. If you've heard of cortisol, you probably filed the information away in your brain next to "black lung" and "Trilateral Commission" as things you know are bad, even if you aren't quite sure why.

Cortisol is a stress hormone, and it's a nasty bastard in many ways. Among other actions, it breaks down muscle tissue to use for energy, the physiological equivalent of using your furniture for kindling because you happen to feel cold one afternoon. And it prevents new muscle tissue from being made.

However: Because cortisol breaks down muscle tissue, you can actually use it as an effective fat-loss tool. I know that sounds like something out of a psychotic economics textbook ("If you spend more money than you have now, the debt payments will force you to spend less money in the future"). But stick with me on this. I've already noted that your body becomes more efficient the longer it does the same exercises in the same way. With this training effect, over time your muscles experience less breakdown from your workouts. That's great for the guy who's trying to gain muscular weight, but it's not the best environment for someone who needs his metabolism to speed up so he can lose fat. About the only good thing you can say about protein breakdown is that it takes some energy to do it. The second-best thing you can say is that it's not permanent. You can reverse it as soon as you leave the gym, by drinking a protein shake or eating something with carbs and protein.

You generate the most cortisol in a workout by doing a lot of work, using your body's biggest muscles, with short rest periods between sets. This type of workout also generates the biggest growth-hormone response. And growth hormone not only helps your muscles grow, it helps your body use fat for energy. The two things don't happen simultaneously. Cortisol causes muscle breakdown while you're lifting, and then growth hormone spikes after your workout, while you're recovering.

So, to review:

- Inefficient exercise causes a stress reaction.
- If you do a high enough volume of inefficient exercise, with little recovery between sets, you'll break down more muscle tissue.
- Muscle breakdown, followed by protein buildup during recovery, speeds up your metabolism, since those two processes take more energy than would leaving well enough alone.

And that brings me to Alwyn's workouts. Unless you've done Fat-Loss workouts designed by Alwyn, your body will have no idea what's coming. Each of the three Fat-Loss workouts in this program has four signature features:

1. *Total-body workouts.* If the goal is to lose fat, then it's best to put all your muscles to work, every workout.
2. *Alternating sets.* No, Alwyn didn't invent the practice of alternating a set of one exercise with a set of a different exercise, rather than doing all the sets of one exercise consecutively before moving on to the next. But he'll be the first to tell you that there are many goal-specific ways to use this powerful strength-training tool. For example, if you were looking to build muscle, you might do pairs of exercises for the same muscle groups in order to induce deeper levels of exhaustion within those muscles. (Shoulder presses followed by lateral raises, for example.) Or to create a more time-efficient workout, you might do a set of bench presses followed by a set of rows, allowing one muscle group to recover while you work the opposite movement pattern. For exercise efficiency, the worst thing you can do is pair up two exercises that have absolutely no relation to each other—squats followed by rows, or deadlifts followed by chest presses. But that kind of inefficiency is perfect for fat loss, which is why Alwyn uses it in these workouts.
3. *Progressively harder work.* In Fat-Loss I, you'll start with sets of fifteen, then go to sets of twelve, then sets of ten. By the end of Fat-Loss II, you're doing sets of eight. (I won't describe the fiendish fat-mashing stuff Alwyn throws at you in Fat-Loss III; you'll learn when you get there.) Heavier weights challenge your muscles more, creating more protein turnover.

4. *Progressively shorter rest periods.* This is what I mentioned earlier as the cortisol-generating part of the festivities. The combo of harder work and less time to recover means less efficiency and, thus, ultimately, more energy expended during and after the workout.

Tell your gut it's time to say good-bye, and let's get started.

Fat-Loss I

Do each of the two workouts six times, alternating between them. You can do two, three, or even four workouts a week. The only rule: Never train more than two days in a row.

Workout A				
Exercise	**Sets**	**Reps**	**Tempo**	**Rest** (seconds)
Alternating sets				
Squat (p. 96)				
Workouts 1, 2	3	15	Normal	75
Workouts 3, 4	3	12	Normal	60
Workouts 5, 6	3	10	Normal	45
Cable seated row (p. 155)				
Workouts 1, 2	3	15	Normal	75
Workouts 3, 4	3	12	Normal	60
Workouts 5, 6	3	10	Normal	45
Alternating sets				
Supine hip extension (p. 115)				
Workouts 1, 2	3	15	Normal	75
Workouts 3, 4	3	12	Normal	60
Workouts 5, 6	3	10	Normal	45
Dumbbell push press (p. 143)				
Workouts 1, 2	3	15	Normal	75
Workouts 3, 4	3	12	Normal	60
Workouts 5, 6	3	10	Normal	45
Alternating sets				
Rotational lunge (p. 185)				
Workouts 1, 2	3	15	Normal	75
Workouts 3, 4	3	12	Normal	60
Workouts 5, 6	3	10	Normal	45
Swiss-ball crunch (p. 169)				
Workouts 1, 2	3	15	Normal	75
Workouts 3, 4	3	12	Normal	60
Workouts 5, 6	3	10	Normal	45

Workout B

Exercise	Sets	Reps	Tempo	Rest (seconds)
Alternating sets				
Deadlift (p. 106)				
Workouts 1, 2	3	15	Normal	75
Workouts 3, 4	3	12	Normal	60
Workouts 5, 6	3	10	Normal	45
Dumbbell incline bench press (p. 139)				
Workouts 1, 2	3	15	Normal	75
Workouts 3, 4	3	12	Normal	60
Workouts 5, 6	3	10	Normal	45
Alternating sets				
Bulgarian split squat (p. 125)				
Workouts 1, 2	3	15	Normal	75
Workouts 3, 4	3	12	Normal	60
Workouts 5, 6	3	10	Normal	45
Mixed-grip lat pulldown (p. 152)				
Workouts 1, 2	3	15	Normal	75
Workouts 3, 4	3	12	Normal	60
Workouts 5, 6	3	10	Normal	45
Alternating sets				
Romanian deadlift (p. 111)				
Workouts 1, 2	3	15	Normal	75
Workouts 3, 4	3	12	Normal	60
Workouts 5, 6	3	10	Normal	45
Swiss-ball lateral roll (p. 173)				
Workouts 1, 2	3	15	Normal	75
Workouts 3, 4	3	12	Normal	60
Workouts 5, 6	3	10	Normal	45

Fat-Loss II

Do each of the two workouts six times, alternating between them. You can do two, three, or even four workouts a week. The only rule: Never train more than two days in a row.

Workout A				
Exercise	**Sets**	**Reps**	**Tempo**	**Rest** (seconds)
Alternating sets				
Front squat (p. 99)				
Workouts 1, 2	3	12	Normal	60
Workouts 3, 4	3	10	Normal	45
Workouts 5, 6	3	8	Normal	30
Wide-grip cable seated row (p. 156)				
Workouts 1, 2	3	12	Normal	60
Workouts 3, 4	3	10	Normal	45
Workouts 5, 6	3	8	Normal	30
Alternating sets				
Supine hip extension with leg curl (p. 116)				
Workouts 1, 2	3	12	Normal	60
Workouts 3, 4	3	10	Normal	45
Workouts 5, 6	3	8	Normal	30
Barbell push press (p. 141)				
Workouts 1, 2	3	12	Normal	60
Workouts 3, 4	3	10	Normal	45
Workouts 5, 6	3	8	Normal	30
Alternating sets				
Dynamic lunge (p. 124)				
Workouts 1, 2	3	12	Normal	60
Workouts 3, 4	3	10	Normal	45
Workouts 5, 6	3	8	Normal	30
Upper-body Russian twist (p. 174)				
Workouts 1, 2	3	12	Normal	60
Workouts 3, 4	3	10	Normal	45
Workouts 5, 6	3	8	Normal	30

Workout B

Exercise	Sets	Reps	Tempo	Rest (seconds)
Alternating sets				
Snatch-grip deadlift (p. 108)				
Workouts 1, 2	3	12	Normal	60
Workouts 3, 4	3	10	Normal	45
Workouts 5, 6	3	8	Normal	30
T-push-up (p. 186)				
Workouts 1, 2	3	12	Normal	60
Workouts 3, 4	3	10	Normal	45
Workouts 5, 6	3	8	Normal	30
Alternating sets				
Bulgarian split squat with overhead press (p. 184)				
Workouts 1, 2	3	12	Normal	60
Workouts 3, 4	3	10	Normal	45
Workouts 5, 6	3	8	Normal	30
Chin-up or Underhand-grip lat pulldown (pp. 152, 154)				
Workouts 1, 2	3	12	Normal	60
Workouts 3, 4	3	10	Normal	45
Workouts 5, 6	3	8	Normal	30
Alternating sets				
Romanian deadlift/bent-over row (p. 180)				
Workouts 1, 2	3	12	Normal	60
Workouts 3, 4	3	10	Normal	45
Workouts 5, 6	3	8	Normal	30
Lower-body Russian twist (p. 175)				
Workouts 1, 2	3	12	Normal	60
Workouts 3, 4	3	10	Normal	45
Workouts 5, 6	3	8	Normal	30

Fat-Loss III

This program introduces a twist on alternating sets called a "giant set." Instead of switching between two exercises, you do four consecutive exercises. And instead of resting between exercises, you do all four in a row with no rest—just the time it takes to get from one to the next. Then you rest for sixty seconds and repeat.

Each workout has two giant sets. You'll do the first one four times (that's four sets of four exercises, sixteen total sets) and the second one twice (eight sets). Then you'll finish with two sets of an ab exercise.

In each workout (A and B), the first giant set is the most important. You want to set up for all four exercises inside a squat rack before you begin. That is, do your warm-up, then commandeer a squat rack, then set up everything you'll need—barbell and dumbbells—for all four exercises before you begin.

The second giant set will be trickier, logistically. Unless you own a gym, or train at some odd hour in a commercial gym and find you have the entire place to yourself, you'll have to move quickly and be prepared for breaks in the action. For example, in Workout A, you have to manage the deadlift off a box, the dumbbell bench press, the walking lunge with side bend, and the cable seated row, back-to-back-to-back-to-back. Even if you set up all four stations, chances are someone's going to hop on at least one of them between your exercises.

That's okay; the key is to set up for those first four exercises so you can get through them without interruption. If you can do that four times in a row, trust me, you'll already be getting an extraordinary workout. The rest of the workout is important to get the full effect, but it's not the end of the world if it doesn't go as smoothly as you'd like.

You also have more variability here than on other workouts. Many of you won't be able to do the chin-ups in Workout B. (I know I couldn't do sets of twelve and ten.) Same with the hanging leg raises in Workout A. I couldn't do two sets of ten, particularly at the end of a grueling workout like this one. If you can, great—do it just as Alwyn wrote it. If you can't, you can do reverse crunches on a slant board (head higher than your feet, to make it tougher than it would be lying on a flat floor) or knee raises on a captain's chair. (It's that thing with the back and arm rests. It's usually combined with a dip station.)

Do each workout six times, alternating between them, for a total of twelve workouts. You can work out two, three, or four times a week, as long as you don't work out more than two days in a row.

Workout A

Exercise	Sets	Reps	Tempo	Rest (seconds)
Giant set with no rest until after final exercise				
Deadlift (p. 106)	4	10–12	Normal	0
Explosive push-up (p. 136)	4	10–12	Normal	0
Bulgarian split squat (p. 125)	4	10–12	Normal	0
Two-point dumbbell row (p. 157)	4	10–12	Normal	60
Giant set with no rest until after final exercise				
Deadlift off box (p. 109)	2	20	Normal	0
Dumbbell bench press (p. 138)	2	20	Normal	0
Walking lunge with side bend (p. 185)	2	20	Normal	0
Cable seated row (p. 155)	2	20	Normal	60
Hanging leg raise (p. 176)	2	10	Deliberate*	60

*Take two seconds to raise your legs, pause a second, and take two seconds to lower them. This will probably feel like a natural pace on this exercise, since it would be very hard to lift your legs faster than that. The key is to lower your legs about as fast as you raised them, which isn't hard but takes some focus, especially at the end of the set, when you're tired and just want to let them drop.

Workout B

Exercise	Sets	Reps	Tempo	Rest (seconds)
Giant set with no rest until after final exercise				
Front squat (p. 99)	4	10–12	Normal	0
Chin-up or Underhand-grip lat pulldown (pp. 152, 154)	4	10–12	Normal	0
Step-up (p. 126)	4	10–12	Normal	0
Dumbbell push press (p. 143)	4	10–12	Normal	60
Giant set with no rest until after final exercise				
Squat (p. 96)	2	20	Normal	0
Wide-grip lat pulldown (p. 152)	2	20	Normal	0
Step-up (p. 126)	2	20	Normal	0
Dumbbell shoulder press (p. 142)	2	20	Normal	60
Swiss-ball crunch (p. 169)	2	10	Deliberate*	60

*Take two seconds to raise yourself, pause for a second, and take two seconds to lower yourself to the starting position.

Hypertrophy Programs

You want to hear the dirtiest secret of the muscle-building business? *Nobody knows what makes muscles grow.* Everyone knows the actions and nutrients and hormonal phenomena *associated* with muscle growth, and for most of us, that's perfectly fine. If I walk into the weight room knowing that the exercises I'm about to perform are *associated with* muscle growth, and that the food I've eaten and will eat *is linked to* big ol' honkin' biceps, close enough.

But at some point, we all hit the wall. We've gotten all we can out of our training programs, and we know that eating more will simply make us fatter. So we tweak things to get leaner, or perhaps put more emphasis on numeric goals, like building pure strength.

That point is when many of us begin to ask the Big Question: What if there's something I haven't tried—maybe something *nobody* has tried—that will make these muscles even bigger?

Toward that end, let's review what we know about muscle hypertrophy:

THINGS THAT GET BIGGER, THICKER, AND/OR MORE NUMEROUS

1. *Protein filaments called **actin** and **myosin**.* These are the microscopic doodads on muscle fibers that actually make muscles move. Myosin filaments are the big boys here, although it would take 10,000 of them to equal the diameter of a human hair.

2. *Fibers within muscle fibers called **myofibrils**.* These are the bits that are moved by the actin and myosin.

3. *Tissue in between myofibrils called **sarcoplasm**.* This is a soup of glycogen (stored carbohydrate energy), fat (another source of energy), loose protein, enzymes, and a few other things I couldn't define or even spell on my best day. One theory I find interesting is that bodybuilders have greater volumes of sarcoplasm than other muscular athletes do, since their only goal is to get bigger muscles as opposed to stronger or faster muscles. In other words, something about the way they train (super-high volume, sub-maximal weights, little recovery between workouts) increases the floating tissue within muscle fibers without making the fibers themselves bigger and stronger. I have no idea if it's true or not, but it could help explain why many bodybuilders (not all, certainly) aren't as strong as they look.

4. *Connective tissues.* Think of a specific muscle—your biceps, say. Connective tissue surrounds the muscle belly (that's the scientific term for "the whole enchilada") and attaches it to your shoulder at one end and your elbow at the other. Yes, you already knew that. But you may not know that connective tissues also surround all the fibers, bundles of fibers, and parts of fibers within the muscle belly. These tissues, like the actin, myosin, myofibrils, and sarcoplasm, get thicker as your muscles grow.

THINGS THAT ARE THOUGHT TO MAKE THESE OTHER THINGS BIGGER

1. *Hormones and growth factors.* **Testosterone, growth hormone,** and **insulin-like growth factor (IGF)** all are stimulated by training and nutrition. They act directly on muscle tissues to make them grow.

2. *Food in general, and protein in particular.* I explain the food-hypertrophy connection in Chapter 21; for now, I'll just say that it takes energy to make new muscle tissue, just as it takes energy to do the exercises that will stimulate the growth of that tissue. If you aren't eating enough food for both purposes—energy for training hard, and energy for turning protein into new muscle—you won't be able to build bigger muscles.

3. *Inflammation.* Yes, inflammation is bad, as a general phenomenon within your body. But, following a workout, some amount of inflammation is needed to make your muscles repair themselves with new protein. If everything's working right, you have a net gain in muscle tissue. Here's what my friend Len Kravitz** wrote in *ACSM Health & Fitness Journal*, a magazine for personal trainers: "The purpose of the inflammation response is to contain the damage, repair the damage, and clean up the injured area of waste products."

4. *Satellite cells.* Another consequence of the muscle damage you inflict during a hard workout—microscopic tears and ruptures in parts of the muscle you can't see and I can't pronounce—is that **satellite cells** step in to aid with the repairs. These are dormant, partially formed muscle fibers (a human version would be somebody born with a head and chest and not much else) that are thought to wake up and attach themselves to active but damaged muscle fibers to aid in their repair.

THE ROAD NOT TAKEN

You may have noticed what I've skipped over so far in this chapter: exercise. Something has to create the damage that causes inflammation and satellite-cell activation. Something has to provoke the hormonal cascade that allows testosterone and growth hormone to do their muscle-building magic.

So let's talk about exercise—particularly, the part of exercise that creates tension within muscles. Back in Chapter 4, I mentioned some of the myths associated with muscle tension, such as the idea that there's a threshold of time under tension that produces muscle growth. (Even if there is such a thing, no one has determined what it is.) But we do know this: Some degree of muscle tension is needed for muscle growth.

For simplicity, let's limit the discussion to **maximum tension**—a stimulus that puts enough strain on muscle tissue to lead to some kind of damage-and-repair cycle. Here are the three that seem to matter most:

1. **Maximum tension created by lifting the heaviest possible weight.**
   If you do a squat or deadlift or bench press with a maximum weight, your muscles are going to be under the most possible tension until you complete the lift. There's also something called **supra-maximal tension,** forcing your muscles to do something that takes you beyond your one-rep max. One example is "negative repetitions," in which you lower a heavier weight than you can lift. Another is "forced reps," which involves having a training partner help you complete repetitions with a weight after your muscles have already hit momentary failure. (Since supra-

maximal techniques tend to be risky and require an experienced training partner, Alwyn didn't include any of them in these programs.)

2. **Maximum tension created by lifting a weight as fast as possible.**

The idea here is that if you push or pull a relatively light weight with as much force as possible, your muscles will have to make some adaptations, even though the weight wouldn't be challenging if you were to lift it at a normal, slower speed. The weight has to meet some sort of threshold of challenge—obviously, you aren't going to build huge rotator cuffs from throwing a tiny baseball as fast as possible. An example is the explosive push-up, which Alwyn includes in the Fat-Loss programs. A push-up is considered the equivalent of a bench press with 60 percent of your body weight. So if you weigh 200 and can bench-press 240, you wouldn't think of push-ups as a serious muscle-builder, just as you wouldn't expect to get bigger pecs with 120-pound bench presses. But if you do those push-ups or bench presses explosively, that type of maximum tension should also contribute a muscle-building stimulus.

3. **Maximum tension created by exhaustion.**

There are lots of ways to exhaust a muscle, but in the weight room we usually talk about three repetition ranges: low reps (three to five) with a near-maximum weight; medium reps (eight to twelve) with perhaps 75 percent of the most weight you could lift once; and high reps (fifteen or more) with a weight that's usually less than 60 percent of what you could lift once.

All of these tension-inducing protocols are thought to have some sort of muscle-building effect. Studies have shown that low reps with heavy weights are best for the most experienced lifters. Other studies have suggested that medium reps create the best hormonal environment for muscle growth—the greatest post-workout surges of testosterone and growth hormone. And one school of thought suggests that high-rep sets can have a muscle-building effect because they create a lot of lactic acid, which has sort of a symbiotic connection to growth hormone. A second rationale for higher reps is that they best employ your body's smaller muscle fibers, the slow-twitch ones, which have measurable, if limited, growth potential.

But you can toss out all the science, pseudo-science, and science fiction, and come up with a much simpler explanation for why different types and levels of muscle tension produce bigger muscles: They just do.

Seriously.

I noted in Chapter 4 that periodized weight-lifting programs—which incorporate different configurations of sets and reps throughout a planned training cycle—produce bigger gains in both strength and muscle mass than do steady-state programs. There's something about high reps with light weights that helps your body achieve the results of heavy weights with low reps. And there's something about heavy weights with low reps that helps you capitalize on whatever base you built with light weights and high reps. Maybe that "something" is nothing more complicated than recovery—giving your body a break from one thing while you work on another. Maybe it's a mixture of your body's hormones and enzymes and growth factors and recovered memories that you can't get from doing the same damned thing every time you go into the gym.

It doesn't matter. Whatever it is, it just is. Do it all, and let your body sort it out.

Hypertrophy I

Alwyn's first muscle-building program has two workouts, each of which you'll do twelve times, for a total of twenty-four workouts to complete the program. (The exception is the experienced lifter training just two times a week. He should cut the program in half, and move on to another program after six weeks.) You can do two, three, or four workouts a week, as long as you never train more than two days in a row.

These workouts are differentiated in a conventional way: Workout A focuses on upper-body movements, and Workout B hits the lower body.

But that's where the similarity to anything you've done before ends. You'll rotate among three different rep ranges. So the first time you do Workout A, you'll do five sets of five reps of most exercises. The next time, it's three sets of fifteen. Then it's four sets of twelve. Then you repeat. Workout B has the same sets and reps, but in a different order.

Your recovery periods, too, will shift around—ninety seconds between sets, then thirty, then sixty in Workout A, and the same variations in a different order in Workout B.

You'll employ supersets for many exercises. Unlike the supersets in the Fat-Loss workouts, which involve exercises that use entirely different movement patterns, the exercises in some of these supersets mirror each other. That is, the second exercise will involve the opposite of the movement pattern used in the first. So bench presses are paired with rows, and shoulder presses with lat pulldowns.

But some of them don't exactly mirror each other. For example, in Workout B, the only superset pairs split squats with step-ups. Both are variations on the same movement pattern, the lunge, although the split squats put more emphasis on the quadriceps, while the step-ups hit the gluteals and hamstrings harder. The goal is a deeper level of exhaustion, for which you'll curse Alwyn at least twelve times before you finish this program.

Workout A

Exercise	Sets	Reps	Tempo	Rest (seconds)
Alternating sets				
Dumbbell incline bench press (p. 139)				
Workouts 1, 4, 7, 10	5	5	Normal	90
Workouts 2, 5, 8, 11	3	15	Normal	30
Workouts 3, 6, 9, 12	4	10	Normal	60
Cable seated row (p. 155)				
Workouts 1, 4, 7, 10	5	5	Normal	90
Workouts 2, 5, 8, 11	3	15	Normal	30
Workouts 3, 6, 9, 12	4	10	Normal	60
Alternating sets				
Dumbbell shoulder press (p. 142)				
Workouts 1, 4, 7, 10	5	5	Normal	90
Workouts 2, 5, 8, 11	3	15	Normal	30
Workouts 3, 6, 9, 12	4	10	Normal	60
Wide-grip lat pulldown (p. 152)				
Workouts 1, 4, 7, 10	5	5	Normal	90
Workouts 2, 5, 8, 11	3	15	Normal	30
Workouts 3, 6, 9, 12	4	10	Normal	60
Alternating sets				
Barbell close-grip bench press (p. 137)				
Workouts 1, 4, 7, 10	5	5	Normal	90
Workouts 2, 5, 8, 11	3	15	Normal	30
Workouts 3, 6, 9, 12	4	10	Normal	60
High pull (p. 181)				
Workouts 1, 4, 7, 10	5	5	Normal	90
Workouts 2, 5, 8, 11	3	15	Normal	30
Workouts 3, 6, 9, 12	4	10	Normal	60
Swiss-ball crunch (p. 169)	3	15	Normal	60

Workout B				
Exercise	**Sets**	**Reps**	**Tempo**	**Rest** (seconds)
Squat (p. 96)				
Workouts 1, 4, 7, 10	4	10	Normal	60
Workouts 2, 5, 8, 11	5	5	Normal	90
Workouts 3, 6, 9, 12	3	15	Normal	30
Deadlift shrug (p. 188)				
Workouts 1, 4, 7, 10	4	10	Normal	60
Workouts 2, 5, 8, 11	5	5	Normal	90
Workouts 3, 6, 9, 12	3	15	Normal	30
Alternating sets				
Bulgarian split squat (p. 125)				
Workouts 1, 4, 7, 10	4	10	Normal	60
Workouts 2, 5, 8, 11	5	5	Normal	90
Workouts 3, 6, 9, 12	3	15	Normal	30
Step-up (p. 126)				
Workouts 1, 4, 7, 10	4	10	Normal	60
Workouts 2, 5, 8, 11	5	5	Normal	90
Workouts 3, 6, 9, 12	3	15	Normal	30
Reverse crunch (p. 172)	3	15	Normal	60

Hypertrophy II

This program is a bit different from Hypertrophy I and III. Alwyn has created three workouts—A, B, and C—that are to be done with at least a full day of rest in between. Everyone is encouraged to do this as a three-workouts-a-week program for eight weeks. Twice a week is fine, if that's all you can manage. Four times a week? No.

The workouts feature more fun with rep ranges: six sets of three, two sets of twenty-five, three sets of twelve, and five sets of six.

Also, Alwyn changes up the tempo recommendations here, which means we'll shift to a numeric system.

In the previous workouts (including the three Fat-Loss programs), Alwyn used "normal" as a default for the lifting speed that feels most natural to you. Let's say you lower the weight for three seconds, pause for one second, then take one second to raise it back up. Numerically, that's a "311" tempo, in which 3 is the lowering, or negative, part of the rep; the first 1 is the pause; and the second 1 is the actual lift.

Here, he mixes it up: 321 (a slightly longer pause on the low-rep sets); 201 (a rhythmic pace for the highest-rep sets); 301 (normal speed, but without a pause between lowering and lifting); and 311. (Even if 311 isn't your natural lifting tempo, try to use it in these programs as your "normal" speed.)

Workout A

Exercise	Sets	Reps	Tempo	Rest (seconds)
Alternating sets				
Barbell reverse-grip bent-over row (p. 159)				
Workouts 1, 5	6	3	321	90
Workouts 2, 6	2	25	201	30
Workouts 3, 7	3	12	301	60
Workouts 4, 8	5	6	311	90
Barbell bench press (p. 136)				
Workouts 1, 5	6	3	321	90
Workouts 2, 6	2	25	201	30
Workouts 3, 7	3	12	301	60
Workouts 4, 8	5	6	311	90
Alternating sets				
Wide-grip cable seated row (p. 156)				
Workouts 1, 5	6	3	321	90
Workouts 2, 6	2	25	201	30
Workouts 3, 7	3	12	301	60
Workouts 4, 8	5	6	311	90
Dumbbell incline bench press (palms facing each other) (p. 139)				
Workouts 1, 5	6	3	321	90
Workouts 2, 6	2	25	201	30
Workouts 3, 7	3	12	301	60
Workouts 4, 8	5	6	311	90
Dip (p. 144)				
Workouts 1, 5	6	3	321	90
Workouts 2, 6	2	25	201	30
Workouts 3, 7	3	12	301	60
Workouts 4, 8	5	6	311	90
Swiss-ball crunch (p. 169)	3	12	321	60

Workout B

Exercise	Sets	Reps	Tempo	Rest (seconds)
Snatch-grip deadlift (p. 108)				
Workouts 1, 5	5	6	311	90
Workouts 2, 6	6	3	321	90
Workouts 3, 7	2	25	201	30
Workouts 4, 8	3	12	301	60
Alternating sets				
Dynamic lunge (p. 124)				
Workouts 1, 5	5	6	311	90
Workouts 2, 6	6	3	321	90
Workouts 3, 7	2	25	201	30
Workouts 4, 8	3	12	301	60
Step-up (p. 126)				
Workouts 1, 5	5	6	311	90
Workouts 2, 6	6	3	321	90
Workouts 3, 7	2	25	201	30
Workouts 4, 8	3	12	301	60
Incline reverse crunch (p. 172)	3	12	321	60

Workout C				
Exercise	**Sets**	**Reps**	**Tempo**	**Rest** (seconds)
Alternating sets				
Close-grip chin-up (p. 154)				
Workouts 1, 5	3	12	301	60
Workouts 2, 6	5	6	311	90
Workouts 3, 7	6	3	321	90
Workouts 4, 8	2	25	201	30
Barbell shoulder press (p. 139)				
Workouts 1, 5	3	12	301	60
Workouts 2, 6	5	6	311	90
Workouts 3, 7	6	3	321	90
Workouts 4, 8	2	25	201	30
Alternating sets				
Wide-grip lat pulldown (p. 152)				
Workouts 1, 5	3	12	301	60
Workouts 2, 6	5	6	311	90
Workouts 3, 7	6	3	321	90
Workouts 4, 8	2	25	201	30
Dumbbell Chek press (p. 143)				
Workouts 1, 5	3	12	301	60
Workouts 2, 6	5	6	311	90
Workouts 3, 7	6	3	321	90
Workouts 4, 8	2	25	201	30
Towel biceps curl (p. 160)				
Workouts 1, 5	3	12	301	60
Workouts 2, 6	5	6	311	90
Workouts 3, 7	6	3	321	90
Workouts 4, 8	2	25	201	30
Upper-body Russian twist (p. 174)	3	12	321	60

Hypertrophy III

Now Alwyn shifts you back to the configuration you used in Hypertrophy I—two workouts—which you'll alternate for a total of two, three, or four workouts a week. Again, you'll juggle three rep ranges: six sets of four, four sets of twelve, and five sets of eight.

The tempos will once again change from range to range, as they did in Hypertrophy II. All of them are a little quicker this time—you won't be pausing at all between lowering and lifting on the main exercises. You'll also do some reps explosively (designated by the letter X on the workout charts). That is, you'll lower the weight under full control—three seconds—and then, without pausing, lift the weight as fast as you can with good form.

And I'm serious about the "good form" part. By this point, you should have excellent lifting technique, which makes it safe to do some reps explosively.

Workout A

Exercise	Sets	Reps	Tempo	Rest (seconds)
Alternating sets				
Barbell bent-over row (p. 159)				
Workouts 1, 4, 7, 10	6	4	30X	120
Workouts 2, 5, 8, 11	4	12	201	60
Workouts 3, 6, 9, 12	5	8	301	90
Barbell incline bench press (p. 137)				
Workouts 1, 4, 7, 10	6	4	30X	120
Workouts 2, 5, 8, 11	4	12	201	60
Workouts 3, 6, 9, 12	5	8	301	90
Alternating sets				
Mixed-grip chin-up (p. 154)				
Workouts 1, 4, 7, 10	6	4	30X	120
Workouts 2, 5, 8, 11	4	12	201	60
Workouts 3, 6, 9, 12	5	8	301	90
Barbell push press (p. 141)				
Workouts 1, 4, 7, 10	6	4	30X	120
Workouts 2, 5, 8, 11	4	12	201	60
Workouts 3, 6, 9, 12	5	8	301	90
Alternating sets				
Dip (p. 144)				
Workouts 1, 4, 7, 10	0	0	n/a	n/a
Workouts 2, 5, 8, 11	4	12	201	30
Workouts 3, 6, 9, 12	5	8	301	60
Dumbbell clean (p. 161)				
Workouts 1, 4, 7, 10	0	0	n/a	n/a
Workouts 2, 5, 8, 11	4	12	201	30
Workouts 3, 6, 9, 12	5	8	301	60
Swiss-ball crunch (p. 169)	3	15	311	60

Workout B

Exercise	Sets	Reps	Tempo	Rest (seconds)
Heels-raised back squat, one-and-a-quarter style (p. 98)				
Workouts 1, 4, 7, 10	5	8	301	90
Workouts 2, 5, 8, 11	6	4	30X	120
Workouts 3, 6, 9, 12	4	12	201	60
Alternating sets				
Jefferson lunge (p. 182)				
Workouts 1, 4, 7, 10	5	8*	301	90
Workouts 2, 5, 8, 11	6	4*	30X	120
Workouts 3, 6, 9, 12	4	12*	201	60
Split good morning (p. 183)				
Workouts 1, 4, 7, 10	5	8*	301	90
Workouts 2, 5, 8, 11	6	4*	30X	120
Workouts 3, 6, 9, 12	4	12*	201	60
Woodchop (p. 177)	3	15*	311	60

*each side

Strength Programs

LET'S TALK NEURONS. I know I've spent the past nineteen chapters focusing on the way lifting increases muscle mass and reduces body fat. But when the conversation shifts to strength, it helps to put an emphasis on your nerve cells, since much of your ability to lift ever-heavier objects starts there.

A bit of physiology:

Your skeletal muscles are organized as motor units. You may think of your biceps, for example, as a single entity that does your bidding when you bend your elbow, but in reality its hundreds of thousands of muscle cells are divided up into motor units—teams of fibers that follow the orders of a single nerve cell. A motor unit could, in theory, be as simple as one muscle fiber acting on the commands of a single nerve cell. The smaller the muscle (such as those in your eyes), the smaller the motor units. The bigger the muscle, the bigger the motor units, so nerve cells in your quadriceps and gluteals could control hundreds of fibers.

When you start a weight-lifting program, your body first has to learn how to do the exercises. It does that by calling in more and more motor units to help execute the lifts. In business schools, it's taught as the "Oh, crap, we need more help here" model.

(Just kidding. I have no idea what they teach in business schools, other than "Pay yourself more and everyone else less.")

That simple biceps curl might involve a weeks-long adaptation process for your body as it throws more and more motor units into action to make the exercise less of a strain on the motor units initially employed. You goose this along by using heavier and heavier weights. As soon as your body thinks it has the exercise figured out, it has to use more motor units because you've made the movement harder.

Finally, when your body has thrown every possible motor unit into action, it shifts to Plan B: making your muscles bigger. That's your goal, of course, but your body is going to do everything it can to resist it. Muscle tissue is metabolically expensive, and your body is designed for economy. You're thinking "Ferrari Testarossa" while it's thinking "Toyota Prius."

The book *Designing Resistance Training Programs* has a chart that explains it this way: During the first week or two of training, almost 100 percent of the gains you make on your lifts come from neural factors. Hypertrophy gradually comes into play; perhaps ten to twelve weeks into a program, increased muscle size accounts for about half your strength gains.

From that point, your size and strength improvements will have a rough correlation. You probably won't gain much strength unless you get bigger, although the converse isn't necessarily true. (It's possible to get bigger without getting stronger; exercise scientists call it "nonfunctional hypertrophy.")

But after about two years of hard and continuous training, added size will be much harder to attain. So, to continue gaining strength, your body will again look to its neural system.

Let me put that another way, and stray from the science a bit to put it in anecdotal terms:

When you're just starting out, you can use more weight week after week because your neural system keeps getting better at performing the exercises. Soon enough, your muscles will start getting bigger, and they'll continue getting bigger as you continue getting stronger.

And then your body hits a wall. It's gotten as big and strong as it can from the standard playbook. Let's say this occurs two years into a program for a serious, physically mature lifter. For a more recreational lifter, it might take five years. For me, it took almost thirty. (I think I mentioned my tragic aversion to squats and deadlifts.)

At that point, in my experience, it pays to focus on strength-building techniques—which is to say, pursue pure strength. It's possible to get stronger without gaining any more muscle mass; weight-class athletes do this all the time. But my guess, based on my own experience, is that most of us aren't *really* as maxed out as we think we are, in terms of size. We've gotten all the gains we can squeeze out of conventional body-building programs, but pure strength is the undiscovered country. For most of us, that new strength will produce new muscle mass.

If you're an experienced lifter but haven't yet hit that wall, you can probably expect phenomenal muscle growth from Alwyn's Strength programs. Let the record show that I'm jealous.

Obviously, these aren't workouts for the meek or inexperienced. You'd be crazy to jump right into weight lifting with programs like these. But if you're one of the millions of lifters who've done everything but focused on pure strength, you're in for a very pleasant surprise.

NEURON DANCE

The goal of a strength program is to teach your muscles to generate more force now, at their current size. Increased size down the road will be a bonus, but for now, these techniques are designed to utilize a couple of your body's methods for getting past your muscles' current limitations:

- Your body learns to "skip" motor units. Normally, when you attempt a heavy lift, your body calls on motor units in order of the size of the fibers. The small, slow-twitch fibers go first, then the medium-sized fibers, on up to the fibers reserved for max-effort lifts. But the muscles of the most experienced lifters can bypass the slow-twitch motor units and go straight to the motor units that contain the biggest, strongest muscle fibers. That allows you to lift heavier weights faster.

- Your body learns to "switch off" the mechanisms within muscles and connective tissues that inhibit force production. Whether you think about it or not, your body has braking systems that it can call into play if it thinks an action you're trying to perform will result in some kind of damage. The longer you lift, the farther these inhibitory mechanisms move to the background. The extreme case is the powerlifter or bodybuilder who lifts with such uninhibited force that he ruptures a muscle or tears a tendon away from the joint to which it's attached. Spend enough time with these guys, and you'll hear stories of triceps that scrolled up the arm like a window shade during deadlifts, pectorals that ripped apart in a sea of purple discoloration on bench presses, and biceps that imploded so spectacularly they simply ceased to exist. (I saw the aftermath of a detonated biceps with my own eyes. It was on a champion powerlifter, and he told me he didn't miss the muscle at all. To him, it was like losing an appendix or something.)

Those two phenomena—skipping motor units, bypassing strength inhibitors—happen unconsciously. You can also employ a few conscious tricks. In fact, Alwyn's workouts employ two variations on a technique called "wave-loading," which I'll explain in a moment.

But the big one, which you can go into the gym and start using today, is called "precontraction." You consciously activate the muscles opposite the ones you plan to use in the lift, and that helps deactivate the inhibitory mechanisms in your targeted muscles.

It's easier than it sounds. On a bench press, for example, you flex your lats and pull your shoulder blades together in back, activating your trapezius and rhomboids (middle-back muscles that assist your traps) before you lower the weight to your chest. Then, instead of passively lowering the weight, you actively pull it to your chest, as if you were doing a row. You should be able to push it back up with more force than you would otherwise.

Wave-loading is another bait-and-switch technique for your nervous system.

In Strength I, after your warm-up, you'll start with six reps of an exercise—squats, say—and then in the next set do just one. Then you'll do another set of six, but with a heavier weight than you used for the first set. Because your body remembers how heavy the single rep was, the weight you use for six reps should feel relatively light, even though it may be more than you've ever used for six reps. Then you do your fourth set with one rep, using a heavier weight than on the previous single. It, too, should feel a little easier than it ordinarily would, since you know you just have to lift it once, as opposed to six times.

You'll try a different type of wave-loading in Strength III: Your first three sets will be three, two, and one rep. Then your next three sets repeat the wave, only with heavier weights for three, two, and one rep.

Focus on the numbers, and look for small improvements from workout to workout. If you make big jumps, you'll probably peak before you get to the end. Your goal is to finish with the biggest numbers. You're free to check yourself out in the mirror along the way—after all, Alwyn has included some higher-rep sets that should help you build bigger muscles while you're recording bigger numbers.

I should also mention a down-the-road benefit of lifting for pure strength: When you shift back to more conventional hypertrophy programs, you'll be able to do six or eight or ten or twelve reps with heavier weights than you used before. And it just stands to reason that being able to do eight bench presses with 205 instead of 195 will lead to a better result.

A FEW WORDS ABOUT SAFETY

I don't believe in using belts, wraps, straps, or gloves, even for the heaviest deadlifts. Instead, I encourage you to do these lifts "raw," using your bare hands (covered with chalk, to dry up perspiration and help with your grip) and your own midsection muscles (to create a natural protective belt).

But I do encourage spotters on the bench presses, and perhaps on the squats. Many gyms have squat racks with side rails that give you a place to drop the bar if you get stuck in the bottom position. That makes a spotter unnecessary.

On bench presses, the spotter should help you lift the weight off the racks so you can take it at arm's length. That accomplishes two things: First, you don't waste any energy. Second, you don't start the lift with the feeling that the weight is too heavy, which can happen if you pull it from the racks yourself. Your shoulders are in a bio-mechanically weak position on the pull, so when you pull from a weak position to a strong one, your body remembers how heavy that weight felt in the weak position.

Ideally, the spotter should be right behind your head. He should let go when you have a firm grip at arm's length, and not touch it again until you've lowered it and pressed it back to arm's length—unless you fail on the lift, in which case he should grab it upon your signal, or before it slowly sinks back onto your rib cage.

If you don't know the spotter, make sure he understands he's not to touch the bar until you give him some sort of signal. No matter what, you've "failed" on the lift if he touches it, so this point needs to be clear before the lift begins.

If you use a spotter for squats, he has to stand right behind you and shadow your actions, all the way into the descent and then all the way back up. Yes, it looks as weird as it sounds. Two spotters, one on each end of the bar, provide a much less awkward configuration.

No matter how many spotters you use, and where they stand, make sure they're strong enough to lift the bar if you get stuck. A safe bet is a trainer wandering around on your gym floor. Unless he's training a client, it's his job to help lifters like you. Another good bet is to ask the biggest, most experienced lifter for a spot. Most of us are too intimidated to approach a big guy, but big guys, in my experience, actually like helping other guys succeed at lifting. There's a slim chance the guy will be a jerk and refuse, but you should be able to tell by his body language if he's approachable or not. Just be polite, and make sure you ask during what appears to be a natural break in his routine—right after he's finished a set, for example, if it's clear he's resting a minute or two before the next one.

One more kind of obvious point: Don't approach a stranger for a spot when you know damned well you can't lift the weight and he'll have to pull it off your chest. That's like asking someone to do your work for you. At no point in Alwyn's *New Rules* workouts should you attempt a lift without confidence that you can complete it.

Strength I

Alwyn created four workouts, each of which you'll do four times. You can do two, three, or four workouts a week, and finish in eight, six, or four weeks. The most important rule: Do all of them consecutively, in the order shown here.

You'll note much longer rest periods between sets, up to three minutes. Some guys can recover in two minutes; others will jump to the next set just because it's so boring to sit around for three minutes. (Not to mention dangerous, if others are waiting to use the equipment.) The key is "full recovery." You have to give your muscles the best chance to lift the heaviest weights on each set of the key exercises. If the wait seems interminable, just remind yourself that it's only sixteen workouts.

Workout A

Exercise	Sets	Reps	Tempo*	Rest (seconds)
Squat (p. 96)	6	6	301	180
		1		
		6		
		1		
		10–12		
		15–20		
Alternating sets (no rest between exercises)				
Bulgarian split squat (p. 125)	3	15**	311	0
Step-up (p. 126)	3	15**	311	90
Alternating sets				
Back extension (p. 117)	2	10	222	90
Swiss-ball crunch (p. 169)	2	10	222	90

*See Hypertrophy II on page 227 for an explanation.

**each leg

Workout B

Exercise	Sets	Reps	Tempo	Rest (seconds)
Alternating sets				
Barbell bench press (p. 136)	5	6	311	180
		1		
		6		
		1		
		10–12		
Barbell bent-over row (p. 159)	5	6	311	180
		1		
		6		
		1		
		10–12		
Alternating sets				
Close-grip lat pulldown (p. 152)	2	6–8	311	120
Dumbbell shoulder press (p. 142)	2	6–8	311	120
Lower-body Russian twist (p. 175)	2	10*	101	90

*each side

Workout C

Exercise	Sets	Reps	Tempo	Rest (seconds)
Deadlift (p. 106)	6	6	301	180
		1		
		6		
		1		
		10–12		
		15–20		
Alternating sets (no rest between exercises)				
Romanian deadlift (p. 111)	3	8–10	311	0
Static lunge (p. 123)	3	8–10*	311	90
Alternating sets				
Good morning (p. 112)	2	10	222	90
Incline reverse crunch (p. 172)	2	10	222	90
*each leg				

Workout D

Exercise	Sets	Reps	Tempo	Rest (seconds)
Alternating sets				
Chin-up (p. 154)	5	6	311	180
		1		
		6		
		1		
		10–12		
Barbell shoulder press (p. 139)	5	6	311	180
		1		
		6		
		1		
		10–12		
Alternating sets				
Dumbbell bench press (p. 138)	2	6–8	311	120
Wide-grip cable seated row (p. 156)	2	6–8	311	120
Lower-body Russian twist (p. 175)	2	10*	101	90

*each side

Strength II

Again, Alwyn designed four workouts, each of which you'll do four times. You can do two, three, or four workouts a week, and finish in eight, six, or four weeks.

The change-up here from Strength I is that, instead of doing waves, you'll be doing sets of four reps on the key exercises, and you'll do them at a slightly faster tempo (two-second descent, no pause, one-second lift). You'll also follow two of your key lifts—squats and deadlifts—with shorter-range-of-motion versions of those exercises. You'll use heavier weights and do fewer reps. Your goal is to be able to do those heavier weights at full range by the time you get to Strength III.

Workout A				
Exercise	**Sets**	**Reps**	**Tempo**	**Rest** (seconds)
Squat (p. 96)	4	4	201	180
		4		
		4		
		12		
Quarter squat (p. 100)	3	3	201	180
Alternating sets				
Good morning (p. 112)	2	8–10	201	90
Dynamic lunge (p. 124)	2	8–10*	201	90
Swiss-ball crunch (p. 169)	2	6	222	90
*each leg				

Workout B

Exercise	Sets	Reps	Tempo	Rest (seconds)
Alternating sets				
Barbell bent-over row (p. 159)	4	4	201	180
		4		
		8		
		12		
Barbell bench press (p. 136)	4	4	201	180
		4		
		8		
		12		
Alternating sets				
Chin-up (p. 154) or Underhand-grip	3	4	211	90
lat pulldown** (p. 152)		4		
		12		
Dumbbell shoulder press (p. 142)	3	4	211	90
		4		
		12		
Dumbbell upper-body Russian twist (p. 174)	2	6*	202	90

*each side

**If you can't do twelve chin-ups in that final set (and almost nobody would be able to), do lat pulldowns with an underhand grip instead.

Workout C

Exercise	Sets	Reps	Tempo	Rest (seconds)
Deadlift (p. 106)	4	4	201	180
		4		
		4		
		12		
Rack deadlift (p. 110)	3	3	201	180
Alternating sets				
Bulgarian split squat (p. 125)	2	8–10*	201	90
Back extension (p. 117)	2	8–10	20X	90
Hanging leg raise (p. 176)	2	6	222	90

*each leg

Workout D				
Exercise	**Sets**	**Reps**	**Tempo**	**Rest** (seconds)
Alternating sets				
Barbell push press (p. 141)	4	4	201	180
		4		
		8		
		12		
Wide-grip pull-up (p. 154) or Wide-grip lat pulldown (p. 152)**	4	4	201	180
		4		
		8		
		12		
Alternating sets				
Dumbbell incline bench press (p. 139)	3	4	211	90
		4		
		12		
Cable seated row (p. 155)	3	4	211	90
		4		
		12		
Dumbbell upper-body Russian twist (p. 174)	2	6*	202	90
*each side				
**If you can't do wide-grip pull-ups for the designated repetitions, do lat pulldowns with a wide grip instead.				

Strength III

Alwyn again designed four workouts; you'll do two, three, or four of them a week for eight, six, or four weeks—sixteen total workouts, all done in the order shown here.

You'll go back to wave loading, with the goal of lifting the heaviest possible weights in the final round of workouts. Unlike Strength I and Strength II, you'll do few sets with more than eight repetitions, making this the lowest-volume, highest-intensity program in the entire book. You'll see longer rest periods—up to four minutes—on the key exercises, and almost every weight you lift will be heavy.

Everyone doing this program should take at least a week off afterward, with two weeks off optimal for many of you. If you do continue training with just a single week off, go to higher-repetition workouts, like the Fat-Loss programs.

Workout A

Exercise	Sets	Reps	Tempo	Rest (seconds)
Squat (p. 96)	6	3	201	240
		2		
		1		
		3		
		2		
		1		
Quarter squat (p. 100)	3	2	201	180
Squat (p. 96)	2	6	201	90
		12		
Seated good morning (p. 114)	2	6–8	211	90
Swiss-ball crunch with medicine-ball throw (p. 171)	4	4	10X	90

Workout B

Exercise	Sets	Reps	Tempo	Rest (seconds)
Barbell bench press (p. 136)	6	3	201	240
		2		
		1		
		3		
		2		
		1		
Alternating sets				
Barbell bent-over row (p. 159)	3	4	201	60
		4		
		8		
Barbell push press (p. 141)	3	4	201	60
		4		
		8		
Woodchop (p. 177)	3	8*	10x	90

*each side

Workout C

Exercise	Sets	Reps	Tempo	Rest (seconds)
Deadlift (p. 106)	6	3	201	240
		2		
		1		
		3		
		2		
		1		
Rack deadlift (p. 110)	3	2	201	180
Snatch-grip deadlift off box (p. 109)	2	6	201	90
		12		
Zercher good morning (p. 113)	2	4–6	211	90
Hanging leg raise (p. 176)	4	4	111	90

Workout D

Exercise	Sets	Reps	Tempo	Rest (seconds)
Close-grip pull-up (p. 154)	6	3	201	240
		2		
		1		
		3		
		2		
		1		
Alternating sets				
Barbell shoulder press (p. 139)	3	4	201	60
		4		
		8		
Cable seated row (p. 155)	3	4	201	60
		4		
		8		
Reverse woodchop (p. 178)	3	8*	10x	90

*each side

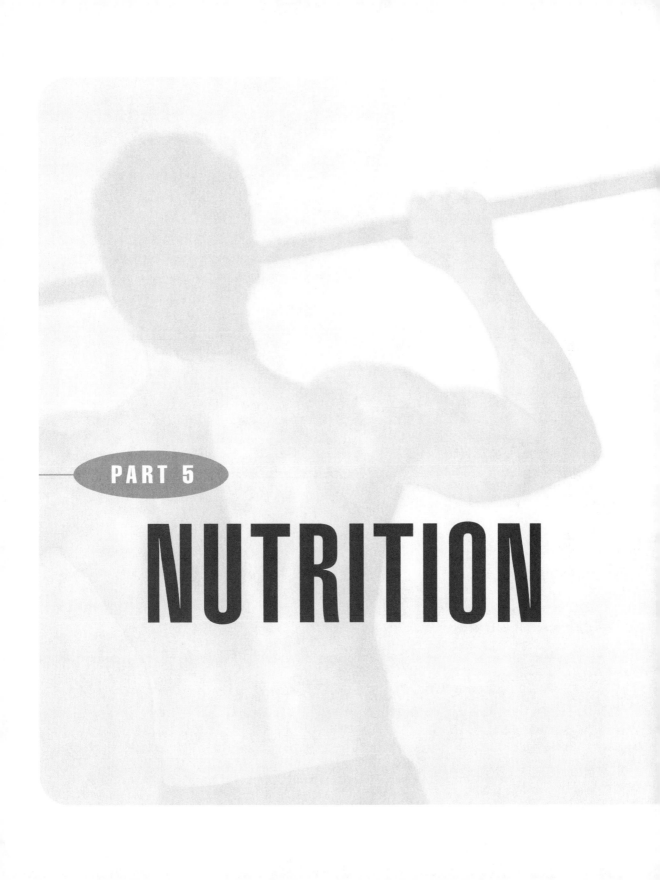

PART 5

NUTRITION

Weight Control Made Easy

I'M AS SICK of the Diet Wars as everyone else. I cringe every time I read about some "magic" food or combination of foods that will produce instant and permanent weight loss. I weep for the people whose weight fluctuates wildly; they go on diet after diet, and they end up fatter and weaker each time.

But nothing makes me more frustrated than the endless repetition of this simple statement:

"If you want to lose weight, eat less and exercise more."

What makes me nuts is the fact it's absolutely true, in the short term. You will lose weight if you consume fewer calories and burn off more. But without a good strategy to cut the foods you don't need and keep or add the ones you do, it's as useless as spurs on swim fins.

Look at it in a business context: If you're a manager and your boss tells you to cut 20 percent of your workforce, you're going to be damned careful about whom you keep and whom you cut loose. You wouldn't send all your accountants packing if that meant you had no one left who knew how to balance the books.

And yet most of the popular diets encourage you to cut calories so drastically that you end up paying the price in your corporeal bottom line: You lose muscle and slow down your metabolism. Downsized muscle and a downshifted metabolism mean most of the weight you regain will be in the form of fat. And, unless you have a metabolism-friendly weight-maintenance plan, you will regain whatever you lost. Plus some, in most cases.

"Exercise more" sounds good, too, until you try to figure out where the energy to do it will come from if you're cutting calories from your diet.

I have two goals with this chapter. The first is to explain a concept called "energy flux," which is a more sophisticated way to look at the classic "calories-in, calories-out" model of weight control.

The second part of this chapter looks at calories themselves: what effect they have on your muscles and metabolism, how to estimate your needs, and how to manipulate your daily intake to lose or gain weight. Then I'll discuss specific foods in the next chapter.

ENGAGE THE FLUX CAPACITOR

Back in Chapter 7, I squashed the idea that you'll increase your metabolism by fifty calories a day per pound of muscle you build. But exercise *is* very much linked to your metabolism—the number of calories you burn each day. So is the food you eat. If you exercise more and eat *more*, your metabolism speeds up. If you exercise more and eat *less*, your metabolism could very well slow down. The combined effect of exercise and food on your metabolism is energy flux. I believe it's the lost key to weight control. It's certainly a phenomenon that almost every article and book gets wrong. If more people understood it, we could wipe most of the popular diet books right off the shelves.

First, some basic physiology. Your metabolism has three components:

Resting metabolism is the number of calories you burn no matter what you eat or do that day. For simplicity, let's call this one RMR, for "resting metabolic rate." That'll save me a few keystrokes. RMR accounts for about 60 to 80 percent of the total calories you burn each day.

Activities of daily living include everything you get up and do, from stumbling to the bathroom when you wake up in the morning to that hour of weight lifting you're going to perform this afternoon.

Thermic effect of food is the number of calories you burn when you digest the food you eat. Not only is it the easiest part of your metabolism to increase, it's the part that most popular diet plans overlook. You have to eat anyway, and by making a few adjustments to your food choices and meal timing, you can burn hundreds of extra calories a week.

Now, a bit of math: If RMR accounts for 60 to 80 percent of all calories burned, then physical activity and digestion account for 20 to 40 percent.

But here's what few people know (or bother to mention): Your daily activity level and food intake have an effect on your resting metabolism. If you deliberately increase your energy flux by increasing your activity level and increasing your food intake, you also speed up your resting metabolism.

The converse is also true: If you exercise less and eat less, you slow down your resting metabolism.

This is the most crucial point I'll make in this chapter, so I want to make sure you grasp it before I move on. Activity and diet choices are linked to your resting metabolic rate. You can increase RMR with more activity and food, and you can decrease it with less activity and food. Clearly, the former beats the hell out of the latter if you're trying to control your weight.

Next:

Most of us know that RMR slows down as we age. A man in his sixties, on average, will burn about 65 calories per hour at rest, whereas a man in his twenties will burn about 75. If each man weighs 180 pounds, we're talking about 1,600 calories a day burned by the older man versus 1,800 burned by the whippersnapper before either guy eats or exercises. So, on average, the older guy wakes up each day with a 200-calorie handicap.

But a University of Colorado study published in 2001 found something amazing: When older and younger men did the same amount of exercise *and ate the same amount of food,* there was no difference in their resting metabolic rates.

The physically active men in this study were mostly doing endurance-type exercise. (The researchers described their weight lifting as "minimal.") Traditionally, that type of exercise has not been seen as having an impact on RMR. But this study showed that diet and exercise—energy flux—do make a difference in RMR, no matter your age.

Practical example:

Let's say you have a guy who wants to lose twenty pounds of fat. His trainer whips out a calculator and shows him exactly how much more exercise he needs to do and exactly how much less food he should eat to lose those twenty pounds.

If it works, fine. But if it doesn't, the assumption is that there's something wrong with the exerciser. He didn't exercise hard enough. He didn't eat a precise number of calories at precise intervals throughout the day. Or maybe the trainer will conclude that the guy has a slow metabolism, the solution to which is simple: Exercise even more, and eat even less.

But a working knowledge of energy flux tells us that the solution is only half-right, which means it's also half-wrong.

Cutting calories while increasing exercise will merely get you to stasis. It won't help you increase your RMR, which is the best weight-control mechanism your body possesses. Think about it: If you can somehow speed up the process that's responsible for 60 to 80 percent of the calories you burn each day, *of course* you'll find it easier to lose fat.

In the past ten years, researchers have tested the theory in both directions. A 1995 study at Colorado State University showed that RMR can be manipulated upward or downward by changing energy flux. Sedentary men and trained athletes had similar metabolic rates when their energy flux was equal—in other words, when the athletes weren't training and simultaneously eating like athletes.

When the athletes trained but ate fewer calories than it would take to maintain their weight—*which is exactly what almost every trainer on the planet would tell a man trying to lose weight to do*—their metabolic rates were no different from those of the sedentary men.

A 2004 study by a combination of University of Colorado and Colorado State researchers provided more evidence of the effect energy flux has on RMR. When older athletes quit exercising for a few days and ate less to compensate, their RMRs declined by about fifty calories a day.

Remember, when we talk about RMR, we're talking about a part of metabolism separate from daily activity and nutrition. It's almost like adding insult to injury: If you stop exercising for whatever reason, and then slow down your spoon and fork to compensate, you still get socked with the penalty of a declining resting metabolism.

But, for our purposes, it's more helpful to look at the bonus that energy flux confers on the guy who *is* exercising. Really, it's a bonus that extends across all parts of metabolism, a universal multiplying effect:

You have more energy for exercise. Scientific publications use the word "energy" the way we use "food." Calories are units of energy. Every calorie you eat is fuel for something; your body either burns it, eliminates it, or stores it. With adequate fuel, you get more out of your workouts—you can exercise harder and/or longer, and that means you burn more calories during the workout.

A harder workout produces a bigger afterburn. I talked in Chapter 7 about the concept of afterburn, the excess calories you continue burning after you've finished your workout. The harder and longer you exercise, the greater the afterburn. Weight lifting, as I noted, has a much greater potential afterburn than does endurance exercise. Some studies have shown elevated metabolic rates for two days after a brutal workout. So if you're working out hard and eating enough to maintain a high energy flux, and then using those calories to help you work out harder, you get the added bonus of burning more calories via the afterburn effect.

The food you eat after a workout increases the thermic effect of that meal. I mentioned that the thermic effect of eating—the calories burned during digestion—can easily be manipulated by several hundred calories a week. The easiest trick is to eat immediately after exercise. A study at the University of Nevada, Las Vegas, showed that the thermic effect increased 73 percent following a weight-lifting session, compared to the same meal eaten apart from a workout. A University of Colorado study published in 2004 showed that regular exercisers have a thermic effect of feeding that's 25 percent higher than that of non-exercisers. That's regardless of the timing of the meals and workouts.

Thus, the power of energy flux becomes self-perpetuating. And it explains why you can get better results from a diet that delivers close to the number of calories you need to maintain your weight, as opposed to a diet that drastically cuts calories.

So now let's take a closer look at the calories themselves.

MUSCLE CHOW

I get asked a lot of questions about meal composition—how much protein someone should eat for this, or how many carbohydrates for that. My honest answer is, I don't know. I can guess, but that's about it.

I can, however, tell you this without equivocation: *Food builds muscle.* Food, in and of itself, is anabolic. Eat enough food to add weight, and you will add muscle. That's regardless of exercise, and aside from all the finer points I'll discuss in this section.

When lean people gain weight, about 60 to 70 percent of it is usually "lean tissue," a category that includes muscle but also bone and everything else that isn't fat. (Anorexics are an exception. They're so screwed up metabolically that their weight gain is mostly fat, even though they're very lean at the start of their weight-regain program.) When obese people gain weight, about 30 to 40 percent of it will be muscle. Either way, there's a mix of muscle and fat, according to a paper by Gilbert Forbes** in *Annals of the New York Academy of Sciences.*

That lean guy trying to gain weight has his work cut out for him. My friend Susan Kleiner** came up with these numbers for an article in *The Physician and Sportsmedicine:* A strength-trained athlete needs 20 calories per pound of body weight just to maintain his muscle mass. If you weigh 160 pounds, you need 3,200 calories a day just to break even—to work out hard and *not lose* muscle. Gaining muscle requires 25 to 30 calories per pound of body weight per day. You're now looking at 4,000 to 4,800 calories a day to add some muscle to your 160-pound frame.

And, as shown in Dr. Forbes's study, some of that is surely going to be in the form of fat.

Is there a way to guarantee that a higher percentage of that weight gain comes in the form of muscle? Probably, although the successful cases tend to be anecdotal. That is, if you tell me your friend's second cousin's training partner built fifteen pounds of solid muscle without gaining any fat . . . okay, I'll believe you. But that doesn't mean I can do it, or you can do it, or anyone not using steroids can do it with any certainty.

One way to ensure the weight gain favors muscle is to exercise, which is so bleepin' obvious that I'm almost embarrassed to mention it. *Almost.* A 2004 study by the U.S. Department of Agriculture showed that, among men, body-fat percentage is lowest among those with the highest daily energy expenditure. (The same wasn't true of women, which should give you newfound sympathy for your wife or girlfriend when she works her rear off in the gym and never actually loses any weight off her rear.)

But, again, none of that makes the case for or against muscle-specific weight gain for the reader of this book, the guy who's lifting weights and willing to tweak his diet any which way to build that muscle.

So now let's look at protein, the stuff of which muscles are actually made. Just a few years ago, the accepted wisdom held that the most protein a body could use was about 1.7 grams per kilogram of body weight per day, or about three-quarters of a gram per pound. Most of us just rounded that up to an even one gram of protein per pound of body weight per day. That means 200 daily grams of protein for a 200-pound lifter.

Your body uses the protein for two purposes: to keep your body from breaking down muscle protein during and after exercise and to help it add new protein to your muscle fibers. I can't count how many factors aside from protein intake go into the muscle-building equation (meal frequency, meal timing in relation to exercise, sleep quality, stress levels . . .), but I can tell you that the ultimate goal is "positive nitrogen balance." Since protein is mostly nitrogen, positive balance means your body is adding more protein to your muscles than it's breaking down.

One study, published in 2001, made the case for increased protein leading to bigger muscles: When experienced lifters were given about a gram of protein per pound of body weight per day, they gained about six pounds of muscle in six weeks. Another group of lifters, eating about half that amount of protein, gained just two pounds of muscle in the same six-week period.

Case closed? No, not because of one study . . . although it is nice to see research confirming the effectiveness of what so many of us do anyway.

Probably the best current information about the interaction between dietary protein and muscle mass comes from researchers Kevin Tipton** and Robert Wolfe** at the University of Texas Medical Branch in Galveston. Tipton and Wolfe believe that the amount of protein you need to put your body into a muscle-building mood is surprisingly small; they've shown it takes just six grams of essential amino acids right after a workout.

But every answer we get brings up new questions. In this case, what the hell is an essential amino acid, and how do I know how many I'm getting in a pork chop, or an egg, or even a whey-protein shake?

Protein consists of twenty-two amino acids, of which eight or nine are essential (depending on who's counting), meaning your body can't create them from other materials. You have to get the essential aminos from food or food-based supplements.

At a conference I attended recently, a researcher mentioned milk as a perfect food for stimulating muscle growth, and it's easy to discover that a cup of milk has eight grams of protein—that information is printed right on the milk carton. But how do you figure out how many of those grams are essential aminos? The answer is three. (Jose Antonio,** a friend who happens to be a nutrition researcher, found it for me.) That means you'd have to drink two cups of milk to get your six grams of essential aminos.

If you don't have friends like Dr. Antonio, you have to look these things up yourself, generally by scanning nutrition databases online and then adding up the amounts of each essential amino acid. If you decide to do this, here are the eight essential aminos: tryptophan, lysine, methionine, phenylalanine, threonine, valine, leucine, isoleucine. A ninth, glutamine, is said to be "conditionally essential," because our bodies can't make it from other aminos in certain highly stressful situations, including major surgery, starvation, and even long-distance exercise. Personally, I don't have that kind of time, so I settle for simply rounding up. A shake mix with forty grams of protein per serving is certain to have at least six grams of essential aminos, and that's close enough for me.

Regardless of whether the amount of protein you eat throughout the day matters as much as we think it does, plenty of research has suggested a benefit to timing your protein intake to coincide with your workouts—either before, during, after, or some combination. (See "Is It All in the Timing?" below.)

If I'm going to err, it's on the side of making sure I have plenty of protein available when my muscles are most ready to use it.

Meanwhile, remember the most important lesson for anyone trying to pack on muscular weight: Food is your friend. Calories matter. Without enough of them, it's unlikely you'll get the results you want, no matter how much protein you eat or how cleverly you time it.

Is It All in the Timing?

The idea that the timing of your meals matters almost as much as their content has taken hold the past few years. And the meals surrounding your workouts are perhaps the most important of all.

Here's the rationale: The purpose of a workout is to shake up your muscle cells, to increase both the breakdown of old muscle protein and the synthesis of new protein. Your goal is a net gain—more protein in your muscles. A meal containing protein and carbohydrates taken right before or right after a workout has been shown to limit protein breakdown and increase protein synthesis. It's the ultimate win-win.

If, however, you wait several hours after a workout to have a meal, you don't win on either end. Protein breakdown continues unabated, and protein synthesis can't happen fast enough to make up for the deficit. So you end up in negative territory, with less protein in your muscles than you started with.

I think it's too soon to tell if it's best to have your protein and carbohydrates shortly before or immediately after your workout. But I do think one thing is abundantly clear: If this is your best opportunity to maximize muscle growth *and* to minimize muscle breakdown, you'd be nuts not to take advantage of it.

COUNTING CALORIES

There is no simple and accurate way to estimate your daily calorie needs. But that doesn't stop me from trying. The following formula is one I've used before with some success, based on the response of readers. To use it, you need a calculator and a scale.

You also need to estimate something I call your "activity factor." That is, the amount of exercise and non-exercise activity you get in an average day. First, place yourself in one of these four categories:

Generally sedentary (desk job, very little exercise, your only hobby is stamp collecting)

Somewhat active (you exercise an hour a day, and spend at least one other hour a day on your feet, moving around)

Really active (your daily exercise involves buckets of sweat, or you lift like a warrior three or four times a week and have the muscle mass to show for it)

Off the charts (you're training for a couple of hours or playing a high-adrenaline sport like soccer or basketball virtually every day of the week)

I've assigned each category a multiplier, based on your age. (Don't worry, I'll show you what to multiply right after the chart.) The idea behind activity factors is that they help you estimate how many calories you burn during the course of a day, aside from the calories you'd burn just to keep your brain and internal organs functioning. I did it as percentages of your weight for a very simple reason: The more you weigh, the more calories you burn with every step you take.

Activity Factor	Under 30	30–40	Over 40
Generally sedentary	30%	25%	20%
Somewhat active	40%	35%	30%
Really active	50%	45%	40%
Off the charts	75%*	60%	50%

*Yes, I had to take an extra-long step in the formula to make it work for the young, super-active athlete. I know some under-30 readers will fall into the big gap between "really active" and "off the charts." As I say below, choose the numbers that correlate with your goals—higher to gain muscle, lower to lose fat.

So here's how to estimate the number of calories you'd need in an average day to maintain your weight:

1. **Step 1:** Multiply your weight in pounds by 11. This is how many calories an average guy would burn if he went through the day without eating or moving. Side note: Isn't it amazing how much energy it takes to keep your heart beating, your lungs working, and your brain generating the occasional thought?
2. **Step 2:** Multiply that number by your activity factor.
3. **Step 3:** Add those two numbers together.

Some practical examples:

Name	Age	Weight	Activity level
Joe Workingstiff	35	200	Somewhat active

His basic calorie need is 2,200 (200 × 11). His activity factor is 35 percent of 2,200, or 770 calories. Add them together and he has an estimated maintenance intake of 2,970 calories. Let's call it 3,000, to make the math easier.

Name	Age	Weight	Activity level
Buzz Hyperball	23	160	Off the charts

His basic calorie need is 1,760. With an activity factor of 75 percent (1,320 calories), his daily maintenance need is 3,080.

However, just a few pages back I quoted Susan Kleiner saying that a really active young athlete needs calories equal to twenty times his body weight just to maintain his current muscle tissue. So Buzz would need 3,200 calories a day, not the 3,080 I calculated with my formula. If I were Buzz, and I wanted to gain muscular weight, I'd go with the higher figure for maintenance, and then add 5 to 10 calories per pound to gain weight.

But let's say Buzz is super-active yet still doesn't have a physique that's as lean as he wants. In that case, I'd advise him to go with the lower number—say, 3,000 calories a day instead of 3,200—and see if that does the trick.

If you're going to be imprecise, always fudge in the direction of your goals.

DIFFERENTIATING CALORIES

I started this chapter by mentioning a statement that drives me nuts: "If you want to lose weight, eat less and exercise more." There's another that I find even more maddening: "A calorie is a calorie." This one isn't half-true. It's wholly false.

Your body processes different calories in different ways. It uses much more energy to digest protein than to digest carbohydrates, and more to digest carbohydrates than fat.

Let's take a closer look at what scientists call "macronutrients," the three major types of food we eat.

Protein

Protein has a higher thermic effect than the other two macronutrients. Different studies show different results, but I think it's safe to say that about 20 to 25 percent of protein calories are burned during digestion.

So let's say you have 3.5 ounces of chicken breast, which is roughly 200 calories. It has about 30 grams of protein. Each gram is 4 calories, so the chicken breast has 120 protein calories. If you assume 25 percent of those are burned during digestion, that means you burn 30 protein calories while leaving your body with 90 to use for muscle repair and other functions.

Joe Workingstiff, described above, needs about 3,000 calories a day to maintain his weight. If 15 percent of those come from protein (as they would in a typical "healthy" American diet), he's getting 112 grams a day, or about 450 protein calories. Assuming the thermic effect of that protein is 25 percent, he's burning about 112 calories a day because of it.

Now, let's look at that same diet with 200 protein grams a day, or 800 calories. (That's 1 protein gram per pound of Joe.) Now he's burning 200 calories a day because of the thermic effect of protein, an extra 88 calories a day. That's more than 600 bonus calories a week. The classic equation says that a pound of body fat contains 3,500 calories, so we can look at these numbers and speculate that he'll burn off an extra pound of fat every six weeks or so, just because of the added protein in his diet.

Does it work like that in the real world? No one knows; human diet and activity patterns are too complex to quantify with simple "Do this, not that" formulas.

Still, I don't think anyone would argue against the bottom-line idea that more protein means more calories burned during digestion, which gives you a higher energy flux. And I've already shown that a higher energy flux means a higher resting metabolism. What's not to like?

Fat

I think it's a good idea to get at least 30 percent of your total calories from dietary fat. (I'll discuss the best types of fat in the next chapter.) That amount supports your testosterone production and leaves you feeling fuller longer—a satiating effect it shares with protein.

One Diet to Rule Them All

If I had to choose one popular diet, mine or anyone else's, as a default plan, something that would help most guys reach their goals, I'd pick The Zone, with its classic 40/30/30 configuration—40 percent of calories from carbohydrates, 30 percent from protein, and 30 percent from fat.

In a recent study (it came out as I was writing this chapter), researchers at Tufts–New England Medical Center put overweight and obese subjects on one of four popular diets and monitored them for a year. The results show that all four diets—Ornish (super-low-fat), Atkins (super-low-carb), Zone (balanced intakes of fat, protein, and carbs), and Weight Watchers (calorie counting, with no major bias toward or against any type of food)—work *when people stick to them*. About 25 percent of the people in each group stuck to their assigned diet to the letter for the entire year.

Average weight loss for each diet, followed by the percentage of participants who were still following the diet for a year (although not necessarily following it to the letter):

Atkins: 4.6 pounds, 53 percent adherence
Ornish: 7.25 pounds, 50 percent adherence
Weight Watchers: 6.6 pounds, 65 percent adherence
Zone: 7 pounds, 65 percent adherence

The two most extreme diets—Atkins and Ornish—had the lowest adherence. The two most balanced or flexible—Zone and Weight Watchers—had the highest. And the people on Zone had slightly better weight loss than the people on Weight Watchers, so if there's a winner here, it's the Zone diet.

And, of course, it's the plan that most closely resembles what I advocate anyway: a diet that is more or less balanced in the percentage of calories from protein, fat, and carbohydrates.

Carbohydrates

For most purposes, I also like to recommend roughly equal amounts of protein and carbohydrates in your diet, simply because it's easy to remember and prevents you from overloading on one or the other. But if you have specific goals to gain or lose weight, I suggest these modifications:

Adding weight: Go for a higher percentage of calories from carbohydrates, especially starchy carbs like whole-grain breads, potatoes, brown rice, and pasta.

Shedding weight: Cut carbs, starting with the starchy ones. (I've also heard them called "dry carbs.") You only need a few hundred calories a day from carbohydrates to keep your body fueled and smoothly functioning; any more than you need and you risk undermining your goal of fat loss.

PUTTING IT ALL TOGETHER

Here's a very simple way to estimate the best diet plan for you. If you did the math earlier in this chapter, you have a rough idea of how many calories it takes to maintain your current weight.

So let's return to Joe Workingstiff as our example. He weighs 200 pounds, and we've calculated his daily maintenance diet at 3,000 calories.

He's decided to eat a gram of protein for every pound of his current body weight. Since each gram of protein has 4 calories, that's 800 calories from protein, leaving him with 2,200 to round out his diet.

If he simply chooses to split the difference, and eat equal amounts of fat and carbs, he needs 1,100 calories of each macronutrient. A gram of fat has 9 calories, so he'll need 122 grams of fat per day. A gram of carbohydrate has 4 calories, so he'll need 275 grams to reach 1,200 calories.

Some people like to think of their diet in percentages. If Joe is among them, it breaks down like this (with numbers rounded off to keep it simple):

Protein: 26 percent (800 calories/200 grams)

Fat: 37 percent (1,100 calories/122 grams)

Carbohydrates: 37 percent (1,100 calories/275 grams)

But let's say Joe isn't comfortable with all that fat in his diet and wants to cut back to a bare-minimum 30 percent of calories. That's an even 900 calories from fat, which gives him an easy-to-remember target of 100 fat grams a day. Now his percentages look like this:

Protein: 26 percent (800 calories/200 grams)

Fat: 30 percent (900 calories/100 grams)

Carbohydrates: 44 percent (1,300 calories/325 grams)

A relatively painless way to put together a diet based on numbers like this is through an online database. I like fitday.com, and there are probably others like it. You'll find that simply tracking your daily calories for a few weeks, and forcing yourself to tweak your meal plans to bring them in line with your calorie goals, can set you up for months of low-maintenance weight control.

Clean Eating

The beautiful thing about writing for an audience is that, at some point, you realize you're learning more from them than they are from you. I hit that tipping point several years ago when I began reading posts on my own message boards about the concept of clean eating.

Clean eating is perhaps the simplest, most elegant way to describe a dietary concept with which virtually every nutrition expert in the world would struggle to find fault: Eat the best stuff available most of the time, and you probably won't have to worry about counting calories. In fact, you probably won't have to worry about a lot of things. Your risk of heart disease should decline, along with your chances of getting diabetes and some types of cancer and the possibility that you'll become impotent. Your waistline should shrink, and your quality of sleep should improve.

Without having a simple or elegant term for it, I described the idea in *The Men's Health Belly-Off Program* when I wrote this:

> You should only eat food that you can picture in its natural, pre-processed state. When you see a hunk of beef, you can visualize a cow. When you see a

salad, you can visualize lettuce growing out of the ground. . . . So what do you contemplate when you look at a Twinkie or a bottle of Snapple? Can you conceive of herds of wild Snapple stampeding through an Arizona canyon? A Twinkie vine growing up the canyon wall?

That's my take on clean eating. If you can't visualize it roaming, growing, or being extracted from something that's roaming or growing, you probably shouldn't eat it. A few good foods take some mental gymnastics to picture: Whole grains, for example, require a visual leap from the hunk of bread or pasta in front of you to the grains that were milled to produce it, to the plants growing in a farmer's field.

You can make a game out of it: Three Degrees of Clean Eating. If you need more than three visual images to get to the food in its natural state, then it's probably not worth eating.

So with the Twinkie, you have to figure out what the spongy stuff on the outside is made of, and then compose two or three mental images to get back to something growing in a field. Then you have to do the same thing for the white stuff in the middle. All told, I have no clue how many steps it takes to get to that wild Twinkie vine on the canyon wall. Whatever the number, it's more than three.

I have just one exception, and that's for protein powders. I need more than three images to get from the powder I mix into a protein shake to the factory that blends it from a variety of powdered things, and then back to whatever those powdered things were before they were powdered. Most protein powders are made primarily from whey protein. I know that whey is a by-product of cheese production, and that Miss Muffett suffered a traumatic whey-related incident. But beyond that, I can't conjure a chain of images that takes me from a cow being milked to the packets or tubs of powder in my local GNC. But I do think this one exception is well worth making; I'll explain why later in this chapter.

I'll start with the foods I put on the Clean-Eating A-List, the ones you can eat every day with no ill effects. The B-List includes foods that are perfectly fine to include from time to time. C-List foods are dodgy, but they're minty-fresh compared with the ones on the Garbage list.

THE CLEAN-EATING A-LIST

Water

WHY IT MAKES THE LIST Assuming the water isn't laced with sewage or polluted with agricultural runoff, it doesn't get cleaner than this. About half your body weight is water (including about two-thirds of your muscle weight), and you can't function without it. Dehydration affects your muscles' ability to contract, your ability to think clearly, and your immune system. A little extra water can help your digestive system function better (especially if you have extra protein and fiber in your diet, as virtually everyone recommends these days). Some research shows a lower risk of bladder cancer and kidney stones with increased fluid intake.

MYTHING LINKS I should add here that I'm as cynical as anyone about the idea that all of us are chronically dehydrated and that the solution is to carry bazooka-size water bottles with you everywhere. Your body has very capable thirst-detecting mechanisms that kick in when your water tank gets a little low. (And I do mean *a little*; they react when your body loses 1 to 2 percent of its water.) And even if you don't react to that thirst the usual way—by drinking something—your brain has special mechanisms called osmoreceptors that sense dehydration and release anti-diuretic hormone (ADH), which tells your kidneys to hang on to your remaining water for dear life.

Another mysteriously prevalent belief is that any hunger you may feel could actually be thirst disguised as hunger. That makes as much sense as a soldier in combat believing that the bullet that just hit his leg is really an arrow in disguise. How long would we humans have survived if we couldn't tell the difference between hunger and thirst?

Finally, the next time someone says you need "eight glasses of water a day," ask where, exactly, that figure originated. You take in plenty of water; a day's worth of food has several cups of it, and you supplement it constantly. The milk you put in your cereal counts. Coffee and diet soda count (yes, they trigger a diuretic response, as does alcohol, but your body still retains most of the liquid). The "eight glasses of water a day" thing is just something somebody made up at some point.

YOU PROBABLY DIDN'T KNOW . . . One of the "myths" that's regularly debunked is the one about how water helps you lose weight. But it's not really a myth. German researchers showed in a 2003 study that drinking a pint of water increases your metabolic rate by about 30 percent for an hour or so and that drinking colder water is better than room-temperature fluid, since your body has to expend calories to heat the water up in your stomach. The researchers estimated that drinking an extra two quarts of water a day would increase your metabolic rate by about 100 calories. Even better, most of those calories came from increased fat-burning. So, assuming your body wouldn't eventually adjust to that increased water intake (as it adjusts to most changes in routine), you could lose an extra pound of fat every five weeks, or thereabouts, just by flooding your system with fluids.

MAYBE IT'S JUST ME Setting aside the myth of massive dehydration in the most over-hydrated society the world has ever known, and ignoring for a moment the interesting and potentially useful metabolic effects of deliberately drinking too much fluid, I think there's a rarely discussed reason why water helps someone lose weight:

If you start each day thinking, "I'm going to drink X glasses of water today," you've started the day by making conscious choices about what you're going to put in your body. I don't know if this is written in any textbooks, or quantified by any published research, but the longer I write about exercise and weight control, and the more experts in the field I meet and pump for information, the more I'm convinced that the real trick lies in planning and awareness. Plan your meals, and be aware of everything you eat and drink throughout the day.

That's the way to ensure that water helps you lose weight.

BEST OF THE BEST Tap water will do, as long as you can trust the source. A green glow is usually a bad sign.

Lean beef, poultry, and pork

WHY THEY MAKE THE LIST The protein is high quality, made of animal muscle and perfectly engineered to build human muscle. Almost half the fat is mono- and polyunsaturated, which are considered very healthy (I have much more on that below). And meat, with its combination of protein and healthy fat, is more satisfying than most other foods. It makes you feel fuller longer, ultimately allowing you to eat less. Meanwhile, the thermogenic properties of the protein help maintain a high energy flux.

YOU PROBABLY DIDN'T KNOW . . . Some anthropologists believe that eating meat helped us rise to the top of the food chain. When our ancestors hopped on the meat wagon about two and a half million years ago, humans became more genetically distinct from our simian cousins. We started living longer, with reproductive abilities that remained intact through most of that life span.

BEST OF THE BEST Go for meat that has the words "extra lean" or "loin" on the package. Those are the leanest, meaning they have the lowest concentrations of saturated fat . . . although it's worth noting that one of the saturated fats in meat, called stearic acid, is actually considered healthy; it helps repair cell walls.

Fish and fish oil

WHY THEY MAKE THE LIST Again, it's because of protein (in the fish) and healthy fat (some of which you find in the fish, although supplementing with fish oil is an easy way to make sure you get enough of it).

FAT TRICK Omega-3 fatty acids, found in fish and fish oil (as well as in flaxseeds and flaxseed oil), are "essential" fats. Your body can't make them from other fats. Again, there's a strong anthropological argument that fish eating was integral to human evolutionary development. And it says something about our modern food chain when you realize there's hardly any omega-3 left in it. Wild animals used to ingest it through the plants they ate, and then wild humans got those omega-3s when they killed and ate the animals. No more; most of our meat is now grain-fed. And even fish are trickier bastards to eat safely, with high mercury levels being reported in tuna and other predator species.

That's why I recommend several fish-oil pills a day (at least six). Each contains a gram of fat, about 20 to 40 percent of which is in the form of EPA and DHA, a pair of omega-3 fats associated with everything from a smaller waist to a healthier brain.

BEST OF THE BEST Wild salmon is considered the best type of fish for flavor, fatty acids, and safety (it's not a predator, so there's little risk of mercury contamination). In fact, a study in *Science* in early 2004 showed that farmed salmon contains many more toxins than wild salmon, including PCBs. But, unfortunately, there's no way to know for sure if the "wild" salmon offered in your local grocery store is really wild. A *New York Times* investigation in April 2005 found that the "wild" salmon the reporters bought in six of eight stores was actually mild—farm-raised. Since the stores were charging premium prices for the allegedly untamed fish, this is a financial issue as well as a health concern.

For supplements, go for salmon oil (look for the word "concentrated" on the label; it'll have more EPA and DHA in it). If the store doesn't have it, plain fish oil is also okay.

Eggs

WHY THEY MAKE THE LIST The protein quality is as good as it gets, and they have very little saturated fat—1.5 grams per egg, which is negligible. (Unfortunately, you can still find nutritionists telling people that eggs are dangerous and to be avoided.)

BEST OF THE BEST Omega-3 eggs, while more expensive, also give you a healthier fat profile. Still, there's nothing inherently unhealthy about the fat in eggs. More than 40 percent of it is monounsaturated, and I'll explain why that matters in the next paragraph.

Nuts and olive oil

WHY THEY MAKE THE LIST Nuts are high in monounsaturated fat, as is olive oil. So are peanut butter and avocados, for that matter. Monounsaturated fat has been linked to lower heart-disease risk, a faster metabolic rate, higher testosterone levels, and lower rates of dementia (possibly because of the vitamin E in the nuts).

BEST OF THE BEST I have a quarter-cup of unsalted cashews almost every day of the year between meals. Macadamia nuts, almonds, pecans, and pistachios all have high amounts of monounsaturated fat. So do peanuts and peanut butter, which are good choices, assuming you aren't allergic to them.

Go for extra-virgin olive oil for salads, less expensive types for cooking (cook at low heat; at high heat, the chemical structure changes). In salad dressings, look for canola oil as a main ingredient.

Multicolored fruits and vegetables

WHY THEY MAKE THE LIST No protein, but their fiber and heavy vitamin and mineral concentrations make them ideal for a fella trying to keep his youthful physique. With different colors come different benefits.

Red fruits and vegetables (red peppers, tomatoes, watermelon) tend to be high in lycopene, which may help prevent prostate cancer and eye problems (macular degeneration).

Orange and yellow produce (carrots, pumpkin, squash) tend to be high in alpha-

and beta-carotene—I know, it's a surprise that "carrots" have "carotene"—which is a powerful antioxidant. Antioxidants—a class of vitamins that also includes vitamins C and E—help prevent damage caused by free radicals, harmful chemicals created inside your body by everything from pollution to strenuous exercise.

Dark green vegetables (spinach, Romaine lettuce, broccoli) have so many disease-preventing properties it's hard to list them all. High spinach consumption, for example, is linked to lower risk of almost every type of cancer. Leafy greens have been shown to lower blood pressure.

BEST OF THE BEST Other than the ones I mentioned, consider pink grapefruit and any tomato products (red); oranges and sweet potatoes (orange); and kale, Swiss chard, and mustard greens (green).

Whole grains

WHY THEY MAKE THE LIST A 2004 study at the Harvard School of Public Health found that men eating the most whole grains had the least weight gain over an eight-year period. That's not to say that whole grains have some magical weight-shedding or metabolism-increasing properties, but there's something about them that helps men control weight. It was a huge study, including more than 27,000 middle-aged men.

ORAL FIBER This is as good a place as any to talk about fiber. It has some obvious properties—helping food move along through your digestive tract, for instance, acting as sort of a hall monitor for your bowels—and some that are less obvious. For example, fiber acts a bit like protein, in that it helps you feel fuller longer after meals. And it also has surprising health-promoting properties. Studies have associated dietary fiber with lower blood pressure and heart-disease risk, although it probably helps that fiber-rich foods usually have the healthiest combinations of vitamins, minerals, and micronutrients, even without their fiber.

I think it's doubly important for weight lifters to focus on high-fiber foods in one or two meals a day, since we tend to concentrate on animal protein and healthy fats. Meat, fish, eggs, and dairy products don't have any fiber, so we have to go out of our way to get it.

BEST OF THE BEST I start each morning with two cups of Kashi GoLean cereal (yes, I'm geeky enough to measure it), which provides twenty grams of fiber. Then, after workouts, I sometimes have an egg burrito made with a Mission low-carb whole wheat tortilla, which has another twenty-one grams of fiber. The recommended minimum for men under fifty is thirty-eight grams, so these two meals cover it.

Oatmeal is another great source of whole grains; steel-cut oats (the slowest-cooking) are considered best, followed by rolled oats. Instant oatmeal with sugar added is considered a poor choice.

Others: wild or brown rice, buckwheat, barley, rye, quinoa. The last one, by the way, is pronounced "KEEN-wah." I actually have no idea what it tastes like, but it's always included in lists like this, so I figured I have some kind of authorial obligation to throw it on mine.

High-calcium, low-fat dairy foods

WHY THEY MAKE THE LIST In the past few years, research into the metabolic powers of dairy calcium caught all of us who follow these things by surprise. It started with studies by nutrition researcher Michael Zemel** at the University of Tennessee. Zemel's team showed that 1,200 milligrams a day of dairy calcium doubled the predicted weight loss of a group of overweight study subjects.

In their most recent study, which came out as I was finishing this book, they showed that a high-calcium diet (in the form of yogurt) produced fat loss of almost ten pounds in twelve weeks. Subjects eating the same number of calories but half the calcium lost six pounds. So, calcium somehow increased fat loss by 81 percent, with total calories, protein, and other dietary variables being equal.

BEST OF THE BEST A cup of low-fat milk has 264 milligrams of calcium. A six-ounce carton of Dannon yogurt has 200. Both of those pale compared with a packet of a meal-replacement supplement called Meso-Tech. It contains a whopping 750 milligrams, along with forty-five grams of protein.

Protein supplements

WHY THEY MAKE THE LIST I don't know if it's too early to say "case closed" about the efficacy of pre- and/or post-workout protein drinks. But I lifted for about thirty years without them and then the past five or six years with them, and for me, there's no comparison. I get bigger and leaner when I use them, and I lose size and gain fat when I don't.

Skepticism abounds among nutrition researchers as to whether protein supplements increase muscle mass over periods of weeks or months, although it seems accepted that they increase protein synthesis and decrease protein breakdown immediately after workouts. One study, cited in the book *Nutrient Timing,* by John Ivy and Robert Portman, showed an 8 percent increase in muscle mass and a 15 percent strength boost in twelve weeks in subjects who had a carb-protein shake immediately after lifting. Those who had the same shake two hours later flatlined—no gains in twelve weeks. (In case you're wondering, the carbohydrates in the shake help stimulate the hormone insulin, which shuttles nutrients into muscles.)

I don't know if that ends the argument or not. As I said in the previous chapter, one lecturer I heard at a conference said that milk should work just as well as any supplement. Since these protein drinks are made from milk proteins, that makes sense. But you'd have to drink a lot of milk (five cups) to get the forty grams of protein you'll find in a standard supplement, which you typically mix with about fifteen ounces of cold water.

BEST OF THE BEST I mentioned Meso-Tech above; Nitro-Tech, by the same company, is another good choice. Both use whey protein, the faster-acting and more potent milk protein. Some supplements use a mix of whey and casein, which is a slower-to-digest milk protein. These include Biotest's Metabolic Drive, Met-Rx, and EAS's Myoplex.

I don't know if there's a magic ratio of carbs to protein. I've read that three or four grams of carbohydrate to every gram of protein is best for pre- and post-workout shakes. My guess is that it matters less than the fact that the concoction contains some of each.

Beans

WHY THEY MAKE THE LIST Yes, they're "the musical fruit," but that's only because of their high fiber content. They're associated with lower risk of heart disease, lower cholesterol, and even lower rates of colon and prostate cancers—there's a lot to be said for keeping the traffic moving down there.

YOU PROBABLY DIDN'T KNOW . . . The gas you get from bean consumption comes from complex carbs called oligosaccharides. According to my friend John Williams,** "We don't have the particular enzymes in our digestive tracts needed to break down these sugars, so they just sit there fermenting in our gut, thus producing the unwanted side effects. Fortunately, soaking them with sodium bicarbonate—baking soda—causes a remarkable reduction in these sugars, and thus less methane." John adds that split peas and lentils don't produce as much gas, so you can spare the baking soda with them.

BEST OF THE BEST The category of beans, also called "legumes," includes peas, string beans, lentils, chickpeas (which sound more festive when you call them "garbanzos"), black beans, fava beans, pinto beans, navy beans, and probably a couple dozen more. They're all high in fiber and vegetable protein. That's not the best protein for building muscle, but it's good for you otherwise.

Berries

WHY THEY MAKE THE LIST If I started nattering on about phenolics, ellagic acid, anthocyanins, and quercetin, you'd think I'd finally gone completely daft. And my spell-checker is already making subtle inquiries about my mental health. But those are just a sampling of the nutrients in berries that make them almost mind-bogglingly healthful. In layman's language, berries fight cancer, infections, and just about everything else that ails you. And some, such as raspberries, are also high in fiber.

BEST OF THE BEST Strawberries, blueberries, blackberries, raspberries—all good, all sweet and tasty, all great in post-workout protein shakes. Fresh is probably best, but fresh berries aren't known for their extraordinary shelf life. (Ours start going white with mold before we even get them out of the grocery bag.) Don't hesitate to buy frozen berries so you always have them close to your blender.

THE CLEAN-EATING B-LIST

Red wine

WHY IT MAKES THE LIST Red wine has a lot of resveratrol, an antioxidant that's also found in peanuts and grapes. Moderate alcohol consumption—two or fewer drinks per day—has been linked to lower risk of coronary calcification, the deposit of artery-clogging plaque on blood vessels. Red wine in particular has been linked to lower cancer rates; one proposed reason is that the resveratrol causes cancer cells to self-destruct.

THIS OPINION SUBJECT TO CHANGE My thoughts on alcohol in general, and red wine in particular, have done a 180 over the years. I used to stay away from all types of alcohol because of the fat-storing, muscle-wasting effects of heavy drinking. Plus beer has boatloads of useless carbs. Plus drinking lowers your dietary inhibitions almost as well as marijuana, leading to the most waistline-wrecking phrase in the entire English language: "pizza and a six-pack."

However, some recent research shows that moderate drinking is an entirely different animal. A little wine can increase your metabolic rate (with the possible negating effect of causing your body to burn less fat for energy), and red wine, with its health-promoting properties described above, looks like the best bet of all.

BEST OF THE BEST I've read in various places that pinot noir made from grapes grown in upstate New York has the most resveratrol, according to research at Cornell University. Pinots from the Willamette Valley of Oregon are comparable, as are French burgundies and Australian pinots.

Average a glass of it a day—and limit yourself to two glasses on any given day—and you should get all the health benefits of red wine without any of the potential health problems associated with too much of a good thing.

Dark chocolate

WHY IT MAKES THE LIST If you have to have something sweet once a day—and I certainly do—this is your best bet. Various studies have shown that it has potent antioxidants and may help lower blood pressure. Even cocoa butter, the main source of fat in chocolate bars, isn't terrible. It has equal amounts of three types of fat: oleic acid, which is the same monounsaturated fat found in olive oil; stearic acid, which is a saturated fat with cell-building properties and no effect on cholesterol; and palmitic acid, which is a saturated fat with few redeeming qualities. Still, two out of three ain't bad.

BEST OF THE BEST It's dark or nothing—milk chocolate and white chocolate are just globs of fat and sugar. Look on the label for "semisweet chocolate" or plain "chocolate" as the first ingredient.

White potatoes and other starches

WHY THEY MAKE THE LIST Potatoes actually rank high on the "satiety index," a compilation of foods that leave you feeling fullest. They have a bad rap because they act so much like sugar once they get into your bloodstream, but that's not always a bad development. Certainly, if you're trying to gain weight, starches help—they provide lots of calories and help stimulate the hormone insulin, which gets nutrients into muscle cells. The guy trying to lose weight is best advised to stay away from them whenever possible.

BEST OF THE BEST The most nutrients are found in potato skins, which few of us eat. As for the meat of the potato—or white rice, or white bread, or regular pasta, or any starch that isn't whole-grain—there's little nutritional value. But, because these starchy carbs enter your bloodstream quickly, they're good for post-workout meals. Otherwise, I suggest avoiding them.

I should add here that sweet potatoes and yams are starches but offer a better nutritional profile. They have beta-carotene, which is why I mentioned them in the A-List under "multicolored fruits and vegetables," and they have more fiber than white potatoes.

THE CLEAN-EATING C-LIST

Coffee, diet soda, and other caffeinated drinks

WHY THEY MAKE THE LIST Given my noted Diet Coke addiction, I'd be a hypocrite if I didn't include them somewhere. Caffeine does help you power up your workouts, with no apparent cost to your health or sanity. And, as I said in the section on water earlier in this chapter, it doesn't really leave you dehydrated.

BEST OF THE BEST Extensive research shows the health-promoting and metabolism-boosting power of green and black teas. If I drank them, instead of Diet Coke, they'd have made the A-List easily. But it's my party, so I'll lump them in with coffee and diet soda, even though any objective analysis would say they deserve better.

Avoid sodas with sugar—it's "diet" or nothing. If you dump a bunch of cream in your coffee . . . well, it's no different from drinking a bunch of cream in any other context. It's almost all saturated fat.

Ice cream

WHY IT MAKES THE LIST It shouldn't, but I like it. So I'll try to justify it by saying that it has a bit of calcium, and at least the sugar is the real stuff, not high-fructose corn syrup (discussed in the "Garbage" list below).

THE INSULIN ADVANTAGE Most foods that provoke a powerful surge of the hormone insulin also create a fast rise in blood sugar. As I said above, when I discussed potatoes and other starchy foods, this is rarely what you want from a meal. A quick rise in blood sugar is good after a workout, so protein and carbohydrates can go to work immediately to repair and refuel your muscles. But at other times, it's the opposite of what you want. A slower blood-sugar rise means a longer, steadier flow of energy.

But some foods cause a big rise in insulin without a corresponding rise in blood sugar. Beef is one, and ice cream is another. (Indeed, all dairy products have this odd quality, although the carbohydrates in ice cream make the insulin response much higher than that of carb-free foods like meat.) That brings me to one of the lesser-known and most underrated roles of insulin: It shuts down your appetite. If you have a fast insulin response, you feel satisfied by whatever you just ate. And if you combine that with a slow blood-sugar response, instead of a quick spike, you retain that feeling of satisfaction longer.

All this may be kind of a stretch to justify including a food I have trouble resisting. But if you must have an occasional indulgence, and I know I sure as hell do, this may be the least-worst in the dessert category.

Butter

WHY IT MAKES THE LIST A tablespoon of butter has eleven grams of fat, seven of which are saturated. So it's bad for you, right? Not in small amounts. Your body needs some saturated fat, and butter has eight different types, including the previously lauded stearic acid, with a surprising breadth of chemical structures. I won't pretend I understand all the implications of that (you don't need to pass any chemistry courses to get a degree in journalism). My point is that your body uses different fats in different ways, and some types—called "short-" or "medium-chain" fatty acids—are preferentially used for energy. That means they're less likely to be stored as body fat. To be fair, I have to say that some of the fats found in butter, such as palmitic acid, are *more* likely to be turned into flab.

But the big reason to be unafraid of butter in small amounts is that it's so widely used as a flavoring ingredient in so many great foods. It's a nice indulgence, and a little certainly won't hurt you.

And, heck, butter falls easily into the category of clean eating. Picture a cow, picture a bucket of milk with cream at the top, picture the cream being made into a stick of butter, and you're right there—three degrees of clean eating.

BEST OF THE BEST Sophisticates who've traveled in Europe and sampled the best cuisines will tell you that the butter over there is different—creamier, more flavorful.

Now "cultured butter" (yes, that's what it's called) is available in the United States, in specialty food stores.

Otherwise, go for "lightly salted" butter, which is best for both spreading and cooking; unsalted butter is used mainly for baking.

Frozen orange and grapefruit juice

WHY THEY MAKE THE LIST They have some vitamins, particularly the vitamin C in orange juice. You're better off eating the actual fruit and getting the fiber (not to mention that by the time you finish peeling and sectioning oranges and grapefruits, you've probably lost your interest in eating), but if it's a choice between one of these and one of the ones on the Garbage list, these are better.

BEST OF THE BEST If there's a difference in nutritional quality in brand-name versus store-brand juices, I'm not aware of it. There may be some benefit to getting OJ with added calcium, although the University of Tennessee studies have shown that dairy calcium has the most pronounced effect on body weight.

Manufactured protein bars

WHY THEY MAKE THE LIST They do have protein. And they taste good. So if your end-of-the-workday choice is either a candy bar or a protein bar . . . well, at least the protein bar has some protein.

BEST OF THE BEST Since protein bars don't fit within any conceivable definition of "clean eating," I won't recommend any particular brands. (Although, personally, I do like Biotest's Metabolic Drive bars.)

ROLL YOUR OWN John Williams offers this recipe for homemade protein bars: "Throw together a bunch of unsalted mixed nuts, dried cranberries, unsweetened applesauce, and decent-tasting protein powder. Shape into bars and bake for about five minutes at 350 degrees, or just until they hold their own weight."

GARBAGE

Cookies, cakes, and other commercially baked foods

Loaded with trans fats, which are now generally considered one of the two most evil foods in the American diet.

Margarine

Same deal: The fat, derived from vegetable oils, is a mutated lipid that is more dangerous to your health than any of the natural ones.

Non-diet soda

Filled with high-fructose corn syrup (HFCS), the other evil food. This very cheap, monstrously plentiful corn-derived sugar is a metabolic nightmare. Unlike other sugars, which your body recognizes as food, HFCS produces such a small rise in insulin that you can drink a six-pack of Mountain Dew before your body realizes you have any actual calories in your stomach. This gets back to my assertion that your body does know the difference between thirst and hunger and also knows the difference between calorie-free water and calorie-rich foods and beverages. HFCS muddies this difference, to the peril of anyone who consumes a lot of it.

Mayonnaise

Store-bought mayonnaise is usually made from soybean oil. Soybean oil is a polyunsaturated fat, and polyunsaturates are often lumped together into the omnibus category of "healthy" fats. However, there's a world of difference between the omega-6 polyunsaturated fats in soybean and other vegetable oils and the omega-3 fats found in fish and flaxseed oil. Research going back decades shows that vegetable oils—corn, soybean, safflower, and sunflower—produce an inflammatory response that's been linked to a bunch of nasty illnesses. Certainly, we have a myriad of diseases that involve inflammation, starting with arthritis and lupus and working up to heart disease and cancer. I'm not saying mayonnaise causes cancer, just that vegetable oils provide little or no benefit and potentially lead to inflammation that could then make you more susceptible to diseases you wouldn't wish on your worst enemy.

However, there's an easy way out: homemade mayonnaise. I got this recipe from a website called cookingforengineers.com: Whisk together two large egg yolks, three tablespoons of lemon juice, a quarter-tablespoon of salt, and a pinch of pepper. Slowly add a cup of very light olive oil by drizzling some, whisking until it solidifies, then drizzling some more. After a few minutes, you have a great-tasting mayo, and you can make it even better with Dijon mustard, garlic, or Parmesan, alone or in combination.

White bread

No fiber, no nutrients you can't get elsewhere, and a near-instant surge of sugar into your bloodstream. What's to like? Williams offers this stark analysis: "For every 5 grams of fiber in white bread, you're getting 141 grams of carbs." In contrast: "For every 5 grams of fiber in lentils, you're getting just under 10 grams of carbs."

Cereals with sugar added

Go ahead and play "Three Degrees of Clean Eating" with Lucky Charms. I can't even guess how many degrees you'd have to churn through just to get the food coloring onto the marshmallow clovers.

Sweetened fruit juices

May as well just swallow packets of sugar. The manufacturers try to dress them up by touting the vitamin C content, but it's really just pure sugar, with none of the fiber or micronutrients you get from real fruit.

Processed meats

Not long ago, we were told that red meat is linked to all kinds of bad things, including the one thing every guy who enjoys his morning "quiet time" on the throne should dread: colorectal cancer. But more recent research has refined that idea. Yes, high consumption of red meat is still linked to colon cancer. But you can get around that in two ways. First, avoid *processed* meat—such as bacon and sausage. According to a 2005 study published in the *Journal of the American Medical Association,* those who ate the most processed meat in 1982 and 1992–93 were 50 percent more likely to have colon cancer in 2001. Another risk factor: a high intake of red meat relative to poultry and fish. (In fact, poultry and fish were linked to a lower risk of colon cancer.)

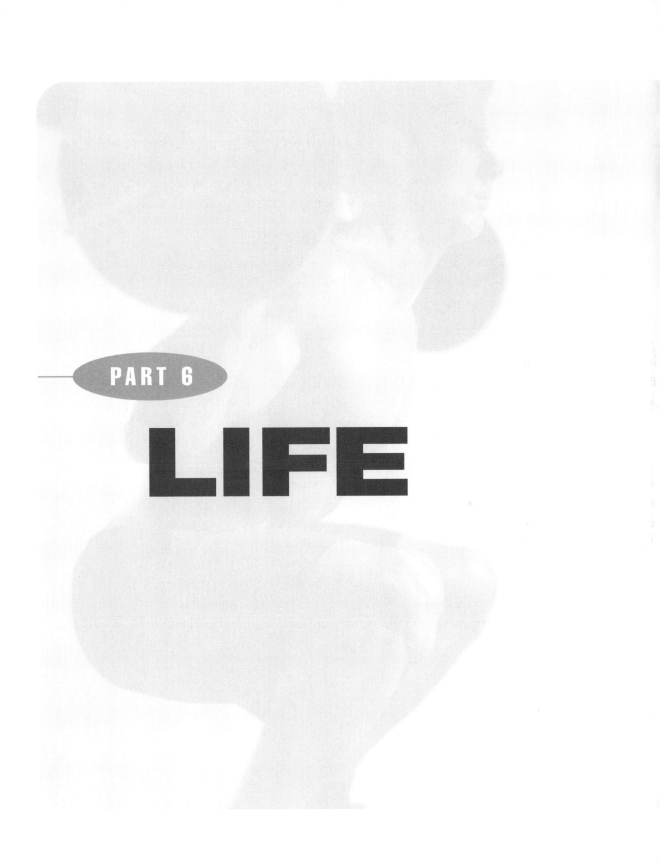

PART 6

LIFE

Long-Haul Lifting

I HAVEN'T RULED in a while, so let me wrap up this book with one more:

NEW RULE #20 • If it's not fun, you're doing something wrong.

A few years ago, I discovered fast lifting. Along with some of the exercises you'll get to try in Alwyn's *New Rules* workouts—push presses, explosive push-ups—I was doing things in which I literally let go of the weights at the top, catching them on the way down. Damn, it was fun. And I never had any trouble clearing out enough room to lift in my gym. Once people see a weight leave your hand, they'll give you all the space you want, and then some.

Not every new technique I try out has that dramatic an impact on my enjoyment of my favorite pastime. But I still manage to enjoy lifting more as my years in the gym pile up.

If lifting hasn't already clicked for you; if it's still something you feel obligated to do, as opposed to something you look forward to and wish you could do more often, I can't predict what the turning point will be.

But here's my guess, just because I've seen it so many times before:

Let's say you go through an entire year of Alwyn's *New Rules* programs, the first time in your life you've consistently followed a structured routine without getting sidetracked. Your body finally looks more like the one you thought you were meant to have, and you're able to pick up dumbbells from the right side of the rack without feeling like an impostor who should be using the smaller weights to the left.

At that point, you feel like a lifter. You're in a gym, you know what you're doing, you're beginning to discover what your body can and will do with the right stimulation, and suddenly you see all the possibilities right there before you. You look at the guys with bigger arms and smaller waists, and you no longer feel diminished or intimidated. You know the secret formula. You've cracked the code. The inches you've gained here and lost there came from the same instruction manual those guys had when they started out—in fact, since you've got the most authoritative and up-to-date edition, you could very well achieve what you want faster than they achieved what they wanted.

I sincerely hope you get to that moment, to your personal clicking point. Maybe some day we'll work out together. If we do, trust me on this: It won't bother me at all if you kick my ass.

Notes

Chapter 1

3   ***Cooper Institute study:*** *Medicine & Science in Sports & Exercise,* October 1992; 24(10): 1080–1087.

4   ***Harvard Alumni Health Study:*** *Journal of the American Medical Association,* October 23/30, 2002; 288: 1994–2000.

4   ***"As little as two months of strength training can reverse twenty years of strength and muscle loss in seniors":*** This is taken from a review study by University of Maryland researchers Ben Hurley and Stephen Roth, published in *Sports Medicine,* October 2000; 30(4): 249–268. I've used this review, "Strength training in the elderly: Effects on risk factors for age-related diseases," as a source in many articles and book passages over the years.

4   ***"More than 50 million trained with free weights":*** This is on americansportsdata.com, in an article entitled "Nationwide health concerns may be pumping U.S. fitness behavior."

5   ***Muscle power study:*** This was sponsored by the National Institute on Aging and published in the *Journal of Applied Physiology* 2004: 96 (2): 814–821.

10   ***Sandow's dimensions:*** I used the descriptions of Eugen Sandow's physique I found in *Houdini, Tarzan, and the Perfect Man,* by John F. Kasson (Hill and Wang, 2001), 42.

11   ***"Death by Exercise":*** You can find a link to this story on my website, louschuler.com (click on "About Lou," and scroll through my bio—a rewarding experience for many reasons).

11   ***Accidental deaths from strength training:*** This comes from "Weight Training Injury Trends," a research paper by Chester Jones, Ph.D., of the University of Arkansas in the July 2000 issue of *The Physician and Sportsmedicine:* "Most of the fatalities were men [31 of 34 recorded in this study], involved head or neck trauma (27, or 80%), involved suffocation or strangulation (22, or 65%), and occurred during the use of free weights (33, or 97%). Two out of three lifters who died were unsupervised at the time of injury. The primary contributing factor in almost all (33, or 97%) of the deaths was unsafe behavior of the participant. For example, one lifter died from asphyxiation after the barbell fell from a homemade bench onto his neck." Ouch!

Chapter 2

14   ***Chek, mate:*** Paul Chek's latest book is *How to Eat, Move and Be Healthy!,* published in 2004 by the C.H.E.K. Institute, chekinstitute.com. For a lot more information, try *Motor Learning and Performance,* third edition, by Richard A. Schmidt and Craig A. Wrisberg. Schmidt's first edition was published in 1991. Editions with Wrisberg were published in 2000 and 2004 by Human Kinetics.

I joke in Chapter 2 about Schmidt stealing my idea three decades before I thought of it, and if Professor Schmidt hears of this book at all, I hope he chuckles at that one. But the bigger concern is that Chek will see the list of movements and think that I've stolen his ideas. And maybe he has a point, since I thought his list was better than mine, and used his.

My original list, which I sent to Alwyn, included the squat, deadlift, horizontal push (chest press), vertical push (overhead press), and pull. I added the lunge and twist from Chek's list and removed the vertical push from my list. (The terms "horizontal push" and "vertical push" come from Ian King, an innovative strength coach based in Australia and my coauthor on *The Book of Muscle.*)

But I want to emphasize here that many of the strength coaches I've consulted in the past few years, and Alwyn especially, talked about the idea of basing workouts on movements rather than on body parts. So this idea was in the ether for a long time before I began to write this book.

Chapter 3

35   ***Eccentric training:*** A 2002 study in the *Journal of Strength and Conditioning Research* by researchers at Ball State University showed that adding some extra eccentric loading to a bench-press protocol improved maximum strength by 5 to 15 percent in trained lifters. (*JSCR* 2002; 16 [1]: 9–13).

However, a 2001 study in *Medicine & Science in Sports & Exercise* showed that going hog-wild with eccentrics, to the point of inducing severe muscle pain, didn't help study subjects get bigger and stronger, and, in fact, set back their strength gains. (*MSSE* 2001; 33 [7]: 1200–1205).

A good middle-ground explanation comes from a review titled "The role of resistance exercise intensity on muscle fiber adaptations," by University of Memphis researcher Andy Fry, Ph.D.: "While not all resistance-exercise programs produce increases in muscular size, most training protocols result in some degree of hypertrophy. . . . It appears that eccentric muscle actions are critical to optimize this adaptation" (*Sports Medicine* 2004; 34 [10]: 663–679).

I also cite Fry's review later in Chapter 3.

38   ***Growth hormones:*** The most important researcher in this area, hands-down, is William Kraemer, Ph.D., currently of the University of Connecticut, previously at Penn State and Ball State. If you're

interested in more information, I highly recommend the third edition of *Designing Resistance Training Programs* by Kraemer and Steven Fleck, Ph.D. (Human Kinetics, 2004). It's among the best books I've picked up on the science behind strength training, and it's surprisingly accessible to non-scientists like me.

38   ***Low reps and muscle gains:*** This study, in the *European Journal of Exercise Physiology* 2002; 88: 50–60, was the first hint I had that maybe low-rep training deserved more attention than it was getting in the muscle magazines.

      Andy Fry's review in *Sports Medicine,* described above, estimates that about 18 percent of the muscle growth in Type I fibers (also called "slow-twitch fibers," these are the ones designed mostly for endurance) is determined by the intensity of exercise. In other words, using weights closer to your one-repetition maximum accounts for just under one-fifth of the growth of these fibers.

      With Type II fibers, the ones designed for strength and power, the weight on the bar is much more crucial. Intensity explains about 35 percent of muscle growth.

      What this means is that most muscle growth can be explained by factors other than intensity (the volume of exercise, the specific program used, etc.) but that there's always a linear relationship between intensity and muscle growth.

      As Fry notes: "[H]eavy intensities must be used to result in a maximal growth response as measured at the cellular level." In other words, you can't get the best possible results without, at some point, using the heaviest weights possible. You're eliminating between one-fifth and one-third of your potential gains when you work exclusively with lighter weights.

      I guess that's good news for the people who are afraid of getting "too big." Small weights help you stay small.

42   ***Ian King split:*** Ian and I wrote *Book of Muscle* together, for which Ian designed three-days-a-week programs, as Alwyn does here in most of the workouts.

42   ***Westside split:*** I wrote about Westside's training methods in the April 2005 issue of *Men's Journal,* which should still be available at mensjournal.com.

44   ***Craig Ballantyne:*** His programs are available at turbulencetraining.com or cbathletics.com.

Chapter 4

60   ***Strength of football players at different levels:*** The study by Kraemer and Fry appeared in the *Journal of Applied Sport Science Research* 1991; 5(3): 126–138. I got the reference and interpretation from an article by Dan Wagman, Ph.D., in the July 2002 issue of *Pure Power* magazine. (Dan is a former colleague at Weider, and he's now editor and publisher of *Pure Power*.)

      I also found data from the study in *Essentials of Strength and Conditioning* (Human Kinetics, 2000), the official textbook of the National Strength and Conditioning Association, p. 309.

63   ***Daily undulating periodization:*** *Journal of Strength and Conditioning Research* 2002; 16(2): 250–255.

Chapter 5

00   ***Warm-up studies:*** *Supertraining,* self-published by Mel Siff, 2000, fifth edition, pp. 161–163.

Chapter 6

73   ***Stretching studies:*** *Medicine & Science in Sports & Exercise* 2003; 35(5): S203; *Medicine & Science in Sports & Exercise* 2004; 36(3): 371–378; *Clinical Journal of Sports Medicine* 1999; 9(4): 221–227. (Ian Schrier, M.D., Ph.D., the author of the 1999 study, also wrote about stretching and injuries in *The Physician and Sportsmedicine* and the *British Journal of Sports Medicine* in 2000.)

74   ***Strength training and flexibility:*** I got this from Kraemer and Fleck, *Designing Resistance Training Programs,* pp. 145–146.

74   ***Spinal discs in the morning:*** Both of Stuart McGill's books—*Low Back Disorders* and *Ultimate Back Fitness and Performance*—are available at his website, backfitpro.com. The former is published by Human Kinetics with a cover price of $48; the latter is self-published and available at his site for $35.

76   ***Pacinian corpuscles, etc.:*** This section is mostly derived from an article on flexibility by Chuck Wolf in the July–August 2002 issue of *IDEA Personal Trainer.* (I also attended one of Chuck's presentations, "Training Movements, Not Muscles," at the 2004 NSCA national conference. If you're a fitness professional, don't pass up any chance to hear Chuck speak. Or just visit his website: 3Dhumanmotion.com.)

Chapter 7

80   ***"Study of nearly 2,000 middle-aged men in the United Kingdom":*** *Heart* 2003; 89: 502–506; two of the study's authors later discussed their results and why they differed from those of other studies, in *Cardiovascular Reviews & Reports* 2004; 25 (6): 274–276.

83   ***"Fifty calories per pound of muscle per day":*** *Journal of Applied Physiology* 2000; 89 (3): 977–984.

84   ***Interference effect of concurrent training:*** Kraemer and Fleck, *Designing Resistance Training Programs; Medicine & Science in Sports & Exercise* 2002; 34 (3): 511–519.

84   ***"Greatest Program Ever":*** *Canadian Journal of Applied Sport Sciences* 1983; 8 (3): 134–139.

86   ***Discussion of energy systems:*** *Essentials of Strength Training and Conditioning.*

Chapter 8

91   ***Bill Starr:*** Bill is the author of *The Strongest Shall Survive,* and he's a frequent contributor to *Milo* and several bodybuilding magazines. He was a national-champion Olympic weight lifter, as well as a record-setting powerlifter, before becoming one of the country's first professional strength coaches when he went to work for the Baltimore Colts in 1970. You can buy the self-published book for $20 at home-gym.com.

92   ***Box squat vs. traditional squat:*** "Squatting exercises in older adults: Kinematic and kinetic variations." *Medicine & Science in Sports & Exercise* 2003; 35 (4): 635–643.

93   ***Muscle use in squats:*** "Effects of technique variations on knee biomechanics during the squat and leg press." *Medicine & Science in Sports & Exercise* 2001; 33 (9): 1552–1556.

93   ***Squats and sprints:*** "The ability of tests of muscular function to reflect training-induced changes in performance." *Journal of Sports Science* 1997; 15 (2): 191–200.

95   ***Bill Hartman:*** Bill's websites include yourgolffitnesscoach.com.

Chapter 9

102 **"Motor-control errors":** McGill, *Ultimate Back Fitness and Performance,* pp. 139–142.

104 **"The meet doesn't start":** "Resurrecting the deadlift." *Pure Power* magazine, September 2001.

105 **"Going Against Type":** "Muscle fiber characteristics of competitive power lifters." *Journal of Strength and Conditioning Research* 2003; 17 (2): 402–410.

Chapter 10

119 **Knee-coordination studies:** "Abnormal knee joint position sense in individuals with patello-femoral pain syndrome." *Journal of Orthopedic Research* 2002; 20 (2): 208–214. "Effects of experimentally induced anterior knee pain on knee joint position sense in healthy individuals." *Journal of Orthopedic Research* 2005; 23 (1): 46–53.

122 **Dry fields and knee injuries:** "Intrinsic and extrinsic risk factors for anterior cruciate ligament injury in Australian footballers." *American Journal of Sports Medicine* 2002; 29 (2): 196–200.

122 **Importance of warm-ups:** "Effect of warming up on knee proprioception before sporting activity." *British Journal of Sports Medicine* 2002; 36: 132–134.

Chapter 11

129 **History of bench press:** I found quite a few historical articles at a website called americanpowerliftevolution.net. The one describing the Canadian Olympic weight lifter (Douglas Hepburn) was written by Terry Todd, Ph.D., who's certainly the foremost exercise historian in the United States, and Paul Anderson. ("The bench press: Part 1" originally appeared in *Muscular Development* magazine in 1972.) The anti-Weider movement is described in *Muscletown USA,* a history of York Barbell, by John D. Fair (Pennsylvania State University Press, 1999), pp. 114–119.

129 **Popularity of bench press:** "Monster Bench." *Pure Power,* September 2001.

131 **Upper vs. lower chest:** "Effects of variations of the bench press exercise on the EMG activity of five shoulder muscles." *Journal of Strength and Conditioning Research* 1995; 9 (4): 222–227.

Chapter 12

146 **Posture and exercise:** "A review of resistance exercise and posture realignment." *Journal of Strength and Conditioning Research* 2001; 15 (3): 385–390.

147 **Superman posture:** This line comes from Owen McKibbin, author (with Kelly Garrett) of *The Men's Health Cover-Model Workout* (Rodale, 2003).

148 **Firemen:** McGill, *Ultimate Back Fitness and Performance,* p. 117.

152 **Old men doing tons of curls:** "Adaptations in the elbow flexors of elderly males after heavy-resistance training." *Journal of Applied Physiology* 1993; 74 (2): 750–754.

152 **No gains in arm size:** "Effects of resistance training on elbow flexors of highly competitive bodybuilders." *Journal of Applied Physiology* 1992; 72 (4): 1512–1521. "The effects of accentuated eccentric loading on strength, muscle hypertrophy, and neural adaptations in trained individuals." *Journal of Strength and Conditioning Research* 2002; 16 (1): 25–32.

Chapter 13

164   *Transverse abdominis:* McGill, *Ultimate Back Fitness and Performance,* p. 11.

166   *Braced abs:* "Effects of specific exercise instructions on abdominal muscle activity during trunk curl exercises." *Journal of Orthopaedic and Sports Physical Therapy* 2004; 34 (1): 4–12. (Thanks to Christian Finn, who wrote about this study on his terrific website, thefactsaboutfitness.com.)

Chapter 18

211   *Stress-hormone response to strength training:* I used *Essentials of Strength Training and Conditioning* as a reference, specifically a chapter called "Endocrine Responses to Strength Training," written by William Kraemer, Ph.D., on pp. 91–113.

Chapter 19

Muscle growth: I mixed and matched from several sources:

- *Essentials of Strength Training and Conditioning,* from a chapter called "Muscle Physiology," by Gary Hunter, Ph.D.
- "The mystery of skeletal muscle hypertrophy," by Richard Joshua Hernandez and Len Kravitz, Ph.D. *ACSM Health & Fitness Journal,* March/April 2003.
- "The science of size," by James Krieger. *Pure Power,* March 2004.

Chapter 20

236   Most of this information came from a chapter of "Neuromuscular Physiology and Adaptations to Resistance Training," in Kraemer and Fleck, *Designing Resistance Programs,* on pp. 53–128.

Chapter 21

256   *Energy-flux studies:*

- "Age-related decline in RMR in physically active men: Relation to exercise volume and energy intake." *American Journal of Physiology: Endocrinology and Metabolism* 2001; 281 (3): E633–E639.
- "Interaction of acute changes in exercise energy expenditure and energy intake on resting metabolic rate." *American Journal of Clinical Nutrition* 1995; 61 (3): 473–481.
- "High energy flux mediates the tonically augmented beta-andrenergic support of resting metabolic rate in habitually exercising older adults." *Journal of Clinical Endocrinology and Metabolism* 2004; 89 (7): 3573–3578.

257   *Thermic effect of eating following exercise:*

- "The effect of resistance exercise on the thermic effect of food." *International Journal of Sports Nutrition and Exercise Metabolism* 2003; 13 (3): 396–402.
- "Role of sympathetic neural activation in age- and habitual exercise-related differences in the thermic effect of food." *Journal of Clinical Endocrinology and Metabolism* 2004; 89 (10): 5138–5144.

258 *Food is anabolic:* "Body fat content influences the body composition response to nutrition and exercise." *Annals of the New York Academy of Sciences* 2000; 904 (5): 359–365.

258 *Anorexics and weight gain:* "Body composition of anorexia nervosa patients assessed by underwater weighing and skinfold-thickness measurements before and after weight gain." *American Journal of Clinical Nutrition* 2001; 73 (2): 190–197. In this study, female anorexics were at 12.8 percent body fat, on average, at the start. After about five months of treatment, they'd gained an average of twenty-six pounds, 55.5 percent of which was body fat. Their body-fat ratios averaged 22.5 percent at the end of treatment, which put them in the normal range for women.

258 *Calories for weight gain:* "Nutrition for muscle builders." *The Physician and Sportsmedicine* 1997; 25 (8): 145–146.

258 *Physical activity and body-fat percentage:* "Effects of the interaction of sex and food intake on the relation between energy expenditure and body composition." *American Journal of Clinical Nutrition* 2004; 79: 385–389.

259 *More protein, more muscle:* "The effect of whey protein supplementation with and without creatine monohydrate combined with resistance training on lean tissue mass and muscle strength." *International Journal of Sport Nutrition and Exercise Metabolism* 2001; 11: 349–364. This study also showed that supplementing with creatine along with whey protein produced even bigger gains in muscle mass.

259 *Tipton and Wolfe studies:* A good roundup of many studies can be found in "Protein and amino acids for athletes." *Journal of Sports Sciences* 2004; 22: 65–79.

260 *Nutrient timing:* The book *Nutrient Timing: The Future of Sports Nutrition,* by John Ivy, Ph.D., and Robert Portman, Ph.D. (Basic Health, 2004), provided this information.

263 *Thermic effect of protein:* "Added thermogenic and satiety effects of a mixed nutrient vs. a sugar-only beverage." *International Journal of Obesity* 2004; 28: 248–253.

264 *Zone diet:* "Comparison of the Atkins, Ornish, Weight Watchers, and Zone diets for weight loss and heart disease risk reduction: a randomized trial." *Journal of the American Medical Association* 2005; 293 (1): 43–53.

Chapter 22

267 The *Men's Health Belly-Off Program:* This book came out in June 2002, to coincide with National Men's Health Week. Although I wrote much of it and edited the rest, my name didn't appear on the cover, for reasons that aren't particularly interesting.

269 *Water and dehydration:* "Myths and realities about water," *Harvard Men's Health Watch,* September 2000.

269 *Water and metabolism:* "Water and thermogenesis." *Journal of Clinical Endocrinology and Metabolism* 2003; 88 (12): 6015–6019.

270 *Meat and evolution:* "Evolution's twist." *USC College of Letters, Arts & Sciences* (a publication for alumni of the University of Southern California), Summer/May 2004. The article cites research by USC anthropologist Craig Stanford, Ph.D., and gerontologist Caleb Finch, Ph.D.

271 ***Farmed salmon vs. wild salmon:*** "Global assessment of organic contaminants in farmed salmon." *Science* 2004; 303: 226–229. "Stores say wild salmon, but tests say farm bred." *New York Times,* 10 April 2005, p. A1.

272 ***Nutrients in vegetables:*** Most of this information comes from *SuperFoods Rx,* by ophthalmologist Steven Pratt, M.D., and Kathy Matthews. If you buy just one book on nutrition, I recommend this one (William Morrow, 2004).

273 ***Whole grains:*** "Changes in whole-grain, bran, and cereal fiber consumption in relation to 8-y weight gain among men." *American Journal of Clinical Nutrition* 2004; 80 (5): 1237–1245.

274 ***Dairy calcium and fat loss:*** "Dairy augmentation of total and central fat loss in obese subjects." *International Journal of Obesity* 2005; 29 (4): 391–397.

274 ***Protein supplements:*** This information is pulled from Ivy and Portman, *Nutrient Timing,* p. 51.

275 ***Beans:*** Once again, I cribbed all this from Pratt and Matthews, *SuperFoods Rx.* Did I mention how much I like that book?

276 ***Wine and metabolism:*** "Meals with similar energy densities but rich in protein, fat, carbohydrate, or alcohol have different effects on energy expenditure and substrate metabolism but not on appetite and energy intake." *American Journal of Clinical Nutrition* 2003; 77 (1): 91–100.

277 ***Dark chocolate:*** "Dark chocolate is healthy chocolate." WebMD Medical News, 27 August 27 2003.

282 ***Processed meat:*** "Meat consumption and risk of colorectal cancer." *Journal of the American Medical Association* 2005; 293 (2): 178–182.

Index

About the Authors

LOU SCHULER is a certified strength and conditioning specialist and author or co-author of *The Book of Muscle*, *Home Workout Bible*, and *The Testosterone Advantage Plan*. A health and fitness journalist since 1992, he has worked as fitness editor at *Men's Fitness* and fitness director of *Men's Health*, and won the National Magazine Award in 2004 for his article "Death by Exercise." He lives in Allentown, Pennsylvania, with his wife and three children, and on most days he updates Male Pattern Fitness, his weblog at louschuler.com.

ALWYN COSGROVE is co-owner, with his wife, Rachel, of Results Fitness in Newhall, California. A native of Scotland, he has an honors degree in sports science from Chester College, the University of Liverpool, and was a European tae kwon do champion. During his fifteen-year career as a strength and conditioning coach, Cosgrove has earned virtually every major certification and has worked with Olympic- and national-level athletes, world champions, and professionals in boxing, martial arts, soccer, ice-skating, football, fencing, triathlon, rugby, bodybuilding, dance, and fitness competition. He is also a frequent contributor to a variety of magazines and web-sites, including *Men's Health* and *Men's Fitness*. More information is available at alwyncosgrove.com.